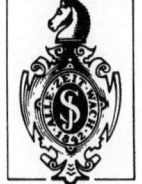

P. D. Coleridge Smith · J. H. Scurr (Eds)

Medical Applications of Microcomputers

With 83 Figures

Springer-Verlag Berlin Heidelberg GmbH

P. D. Coleridge Smith, MA, BM, FRCS
Senior Lecturer in Surgical Science, Department of Surgical
Studies, University College and Middlesex School of Medicine,
Mortimer Street, London W1N 8AA, UK.

J. H. Scurr, BSc, FRCS
Senior Lecturer in Surgery and Honorary Consultant Surgeon,
Department of Surgical Studies, University College and Middlesex
School of Medicine, Mortimer Street, London W1N 8AA, UK.

ISBN 978-1-4471-1663-9   ISBN 978-1-4471-1661-5 (eBook)
DOI 10.1007/978-1-4471-1661-5

British Library Catologuing in Pubication Data
Medical applications of microcomputers.
1. Medicine. Applications of microcomputer systems
I. Coleridge Smith, P.D. (Philip David), *1953—*
II. Scurr, J.H. (John Henry), *1947—*
610'.28'5416
ISBN 978-1-4471-1663-9

Library of Congress Cataloging-in-Publication Data
Medical applications of microcomputers.
"Proceedings of the Fifth Medical Microcomputer Applications Workshop which was
held at the Middlesex Hospital on 1 and 2, October 1987"—Pref.
  Includes bibliographies and index.
  1. Medicine, Clinical—Data processing—Congresses. 2. Microcomputers—Con-
gresses. I. Coleridge Smith, P. D. (Philip David), 1953—   . II. Scurr, J. H. (John
Henry), 1947—   . III. Medical Microcomputer Applications Workshop (5th: 1987:
Middlesex Hospital)
[DNLM: 1. Computers—congresses. W 26.5 M4886 1987]
R858.A2M38 1988 616.075 88-24841
ISBN 978-1-4471-1663-9

© Springer-Verlag Berlin Heidelberg 1988
Originally published by Springer-Verlag Berlin Heidelberg New York in 1988
Softcover reprint of the hardcover 1st edition 1988

Filmset by Wilmaset, Birkenhead, Wirral

2128/3916-543210—Printed on acid-free paper

Preface

This book is based on the proceedings of the fifth Medical Micro-computer Applications Workshop which was held at the Middlesex Hospital on 1 and 2 October 1987. The meeting was attended by clinicians from many disciplines, and by computer scientists and engineers. Discussions centred on many areas of clinical practice in which microcomputers are being used. Advances in microcomputer technology are reflected in the projects described, including the use of local area networks and applications involving 16-bit microcomputers. Applications involving IBM-compatible microcomputers and Apple Macintosh machines are described. A wide range of clinical applications are presented including the recording of patient data, combined with powerful data-processing facilities permitting the construction of clinical audit systems. In further applications the computer obtains and analyses physiological data directly from transducers attached to the patient. A variety of clinical management systems involving microcomputers are described. Some advise the clinician on patient management, and others have the capability to administer a drug in a variable dose based on directly measured physiological parameters.

The ingenuity and imagination of the authors who describe their work in this book has been applied to their own areas in medicine. This indicates what may be achieved by clinicians who have both a wide interest in their subject and an understanding of microcomputer applications. The projects described here illustrate some of the capabilities of microcomputers in medicine at the present time, and indicate possible areas for further advances. These depend on micro-computer advances now taking place, including the development of expert systems and image processing capabilities.

Strict controls are necessary to prevent computers from adversely affecting patient management. Errors in audit systems may provide misleading information adversely affecting future planning. Software

and hardware errors may lead to data corruption and the systems that
we develop require built-in checks for these problems, particularly
when the computer is directly responsible for drug administration.
This problem is addressed by those authors whose systems have the
capability directly to alter patient treatment.

We expect that this book will be a useful source of information on
techniques and programming methods for readers wishing to
implement their own medical microcomputer applications.

The Middlesex Hospital, London W1   P. D. Coleridge Smith
March 1988   J. H. Scurr

Contents

Contributors

Hilary A. Aitken
Research Registrar, University Department of Anaesthesia,
Glasgow Royal Infirmary, Glasgow G31 2ER

R. E. Ashton
Consultant Dermatologist, Royal Navy Hospital, Haslar, Gosport,
Hampshire

C. Bloor
Senior Lecturer in Computer Studies, School of Computer Studies
and Mathematics, Sunderland Polytechnic, Priestman Building,
Green Terrace, Sunderland SR1 3SD

G. Boran
Registrar, Department of Chemical Pathology and Human
Metabolism, Royal Free Hospital, Pond Street, London NW3 2QG

G. J. Brooks
Royal Naval Medical Officer, On attachment to Department of
Medical Informatics and Computing, Pond Street, London NW3
2QG

D. Bryce
Analyst Programmer, University Computing Services (Medical
Unit), Ninewells Hospital & Medical School, Dundee DD1 9SY

C. Carey
Medical Registrar, Department of Cardiology, The London
Hospital, Whitechapel Road, London EC1

N. W. Carter
Director, Medical Computer Unit, University Computing Services
(Medical Unit), Ninewells Hospital & Medical School, Dundee
DD1 9SY

C. R. Chapple
Senior Registrar, Department of Urology, The Middlesex Hospital,
London W1N 8AA

P. O. Collinson
Senior Registrar, Department of Clinical Biochemistry, West
Middlesex University Hospital, Isleworth, Middlesex TW7 6AF

J. R. Colvin
Research Registrar, University Department of Anaesthesia,
Glasgow Royal Infirmary, Glasgow G31 2ER

I. C. Cooper
Senior Registrar, Department of Cardiology, St Thomas' Hospital,
Lambeth Palace Road, London SE1 7EH

D. Cramp
Senior Lecturer, Department of Medical Informatics, Royal Free
Hospital School of Medicine, Pond Street, London NW3 2QG

A. Crowther
Chief Technician
Department of Cardiology, St Thomas' Hospital, Lambeth Palace
Road, London SE1 7EH

C. J. de Gara
Surgical Registrar, The Bloomsbury Breast Clinic, University
College Hospital, Gower Street, London WC1

O. H. B. Gyde
Consultant Haematologist, Department of Haematology, East
Birmingham Hospital, Bordesley Green East, Birmingham B9 5ST

K. E. F. Hobbs
Professor of Surgery, Academic Department of Surgery, Royal
Free Hospital School of Medicine, Pond Street, London NW3 2QG

M. Howes
Lecturer, Department of Psychology, University of Leeds, Leeds

S. W. Hughes
Senior Physicist, Department of Medical Physics, St Thomas'
Hospital, Lambeth Palace Road, London SE1 7EH

R. G. Jones
Senior Registrar, Department of Chemical Pathology, St James's
University Hospital, Beckett Street, Leeds LS9 7TF

D. Katritsis
Research Registrar
Department of Cardiology, St Thomas' Hospital, Lambeth Palace
Road, London SE1 7EH

G. N. C. Kenny
Senior Lecturer in Anaesthesia, University Department of
Anaesthesia, Glasgow Royal Infirmary, Glasgow G31 2ER

B. E. Keogh
British Heart Foundation Research Fellow in Cardiac Surgery,
Department of Cardiac Surgery, Royal Postgraduate Medical
School, Du Cane Road, London W12 OHS

J. G. Malone-Lee
Senior Lecturer in Geriatric Medicine, Academic Department of
Geriatric Medicine, University College Hospital, Gower Street,
London WC1

C. S. McArdle
Consultant Surgeon, University Department of Anaesthesia,
Glasgow Royal Infirmary, Glasgow G31 2ER

R. J. Pethybridge
Statistician, Royal Navy Hospital Haslar and Institute of Naval
Medicine, Gosport, Hampshire

K. Renner
Senior Physiological Technician, Department of Cardiology, The
Royal Sussex County Hospital, Eastern Road, Brighton BN2 5BE

J. E. Saunders
Chief Physicist, Department of Medical Physics, St Thomas'
Hospital, Lambeth Palace Road, London SE1 7EH

J. H. Scurr
Consultant Surgeon, The Bloomsbury Breast Clinic, University
College Hospital, Gower Street, London WC1

A. M. Seifalian
Senior Biophysicist, Academic Department of Surgery, Royal Free
Hospital School of Medicine, Pond Street, London NW3 2QG

J. L. Shearer
Analyst Programmer, University Computing Services (Medical
Unit), Ninewells Hospital and Medical School, Dundee DD1 9SY

A. R. Timothy
Consultant Radiotherapist, Department of Radiotherapy, St
Thomas' Hospital, Lambeth Palace Road, London SE1 7EH

R. L. Vaghjiani
Computer Scientist, Department of Medical Physics, The Royal
Free Hospital, Pond Street, London NW3 2QG

M. A. Walker
Surgical Registrar, Department of Surgery, Ninewells Hospital &
Medical School, Dundee DD1 9SY

N. Watson
Consultant Hand and Orthopaedic Surgeon, Milton Keynes District
Hospital, Milton Keynes MK6 5LR

M. M. Webb-Peploe
Consultant Cardiologist, Department of Cardiology, St Thomas'
Hospital, Lambeth Palace Road, London SE1 7EH

R. J. Whiddett
Head of Microcomputer Unit, Department of Computing,
University of Lancaster, Bailrigg, Lancaster, LA1 4YR

1 Information Management for Breast Clinics

C.J. de Gara and J.H. Scurr

Introduction

Breast disease is common with 16% of all women seeking surgical advice (Nicols, Waters and Wheeler 1980), while benign breast disease may affect up to 50% of women (Haagenson 1971). Public awareness of the breast cancer risk of 1:17 with an annual incidence of 50–200:100 000 (Pike et al. 1983) has increased attendance rates in surgical clinics and promoted the development of specialist breast clinics.

The Bloomsbury Breast Clinic has evolved to service this requirement and currently sees 30–35 newly referred and 60–80 follow-up patients per week. Since breast disease presents limited diagnostic and management options, computerisation provides a logical enhancement to current clinical practice. Despite the obvious advantages of rapid, easy and accurate storage, retrieval and analysis of patient data, microcomputers continue to be viewed by the medical profession as principally research tools. In part, the problem is one of a lack of universal policy throughout the National Health Service, but there is also a general experience of failure of earlier systems. These failures frequently occurred because of excessive complexity, limited direct clinical benefits and reliance on non-keyboard-competent individuals (usually busy doctors) entering data.

The aim of the Bloomsbury Breast Clinic Information Management System was to create a microcomputer-based set-up which would take over many of the routine tasks performed by the clinic secretary, such as letter writing and searching for investigation results, and which would avoid the need for medical staff to enter patient information. Additionally, with improved patient data storage, the potentially serious but common problem of lost or unobtainable patient notes should not occur.

Hardware and Software Consideration

Accepting certain limitations of commercially available software the system was developed using DataEase version 2.5 (Sapphire Systems Limited, UK) a menu driven, relational, fourth generation programming language database. This database is capable of 255 fields per record, 65 535 records per file with 28 files open concurrently. In order to run a database of this size and complexity an IBM AT compatible, a Tandon PCA 20 (286 CPU running at 8 MHz with a 20 Mbyte hard disc) was employed.

Database Structure

Central to the structure of the database was the concept that patients attending a breast clinic fall into one of five categories (forms):

1. New patients (new referrals)
2. Second visit (next attendance following referral)
3. Ex in-patient (attendance following admission)
4. Benign follow-up (attendance(s) for benign disease)
5. Cancer follow-up (attendance(s) for breast cancer)

Linking these categories in a relational manner is the demographic data (name, hospital number, age, address, GP details) or Patient Details form.

Data Collection

Each form contains a different number of fields pertaining to history, examination, diagnosis and treatment (Patient Details = 24, New Pt = 112, Second Visit = 63, Ex In Pt = 38, Benign FU = 93, Ca FU = 97). These fields were defined when the overall structure of the database was designed. At that time fields were designated as being either numeric (e.g. number of months of symptoms), date (e.g. date of birth, attendance, last menstrual period), yes/no, choice (e.g. nipple discharge clear/blood-stained/yellow/milky), calculated (e.g. age) or text (e.g. histology, mammography or cytology report). Patient name and hospital number are indexed to speed up record searches. Colour-coded hard copy sheets of each form are used in the clinic and completed by the doctor during the patient interview and examination. These single colour sheets have exactly the same field layout as well as all field options listed. Completing the sheet is a simple matter of ringing the relevant field options i.e. selecting the diagnosis from a choice of 15 listed. Four lines for free text comment are available at the end of each sheet and that comment will subsequently be incorporated into the GP letter. Reports from

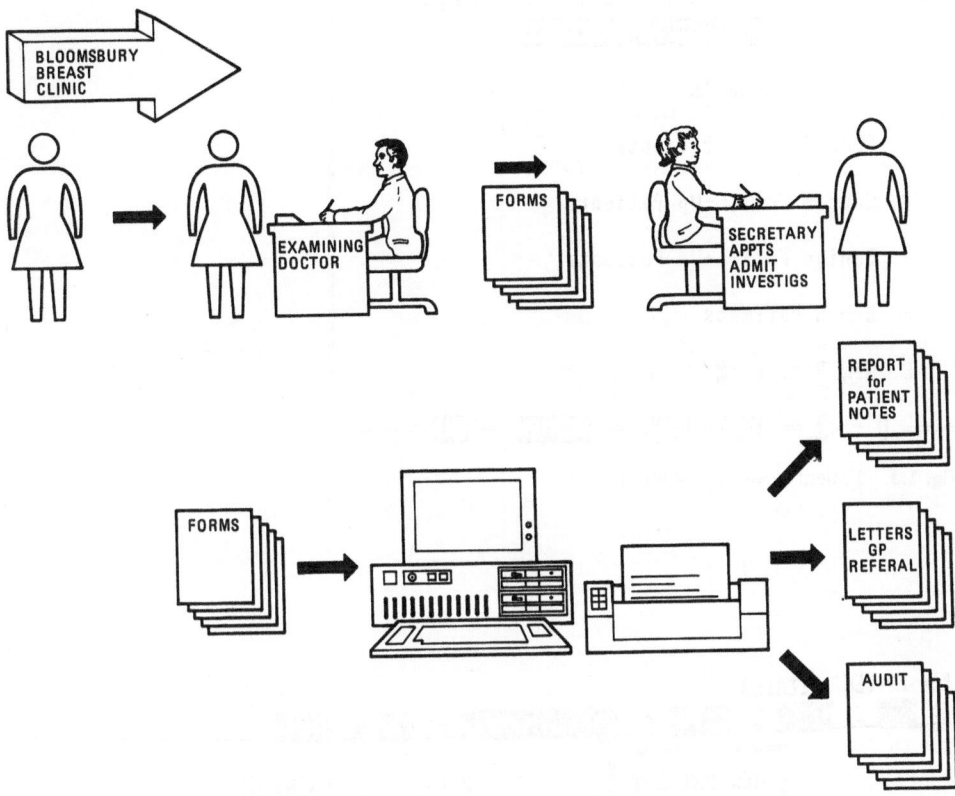

Fig. 1.1. Scheme of the Bloomsbury Breast Clinic Information Management System.

THE BLOOMSBURY BREAST CLINIC

1. Patient Record Entry

2. Patient Letters

3. DNA Letters

4. Audit

5. Print Clinic Lists

6. Print Patient Records

1 to 6 = UP = DOWN = RETURN = END

Fig. 1.2. Main menu of available options within system.

```
┌─────────────────────────────────────────────┐
│           PATIENT RECORD ENTRY                │
│                                               │
│     1. Patient Details                        │
│                                               │
│     2. Second Visit Patients                  │
│                                               │
│     3. Cancer Follow-Up Patients              │
│                                               │
│     4. Benign Follow-Up Patients              │
│                                               │
│     5. Ex-In Patients                         │
│                                               │
│     6. New Patients                           │
└─────────────────────────────────────────────┘
═══ 1 to 3 ═ UP ═ DOWN ═ RETURN ═ END ═══
```

Fig. 1.3. Patient record entry menu.

NEW PATIENT DETAILS
1: None 2: Milky 3: Clear 4: Blood Stained 5: Pus 6: Green

```
         ┌──────────────┐        Date    : 08/01/87
         │ NEW PATIENT  │        Seen by : Registrar, Mr de Gara
         └──────────────┘
Name : ███████████████████████   Hosp No.  89-15
```

```
         ┌──────────┐
         │ HISTORY  │
         └──────────┘
```

Lump yes Observer Self_____ Side Left_ Duration __6(weeks) Painful yes

Mastalgia None_____ Side Both_ Duration __6_ (weeks)

Nipple Discharge None_____ Side ____ Duration ___(weeks)

Nipple Change no_ Side ____ Duration ___(weeks)

F2 ENTER F3 VIEW F4 EXIT F5 FORM CLR F6 FLD CLR F7 DELETE F8 MODIFY F9 REPORT F10 MULTI

Fig. 1.4. Example of New Patient Form as seen on the computer screen showing the first of 6 screens.

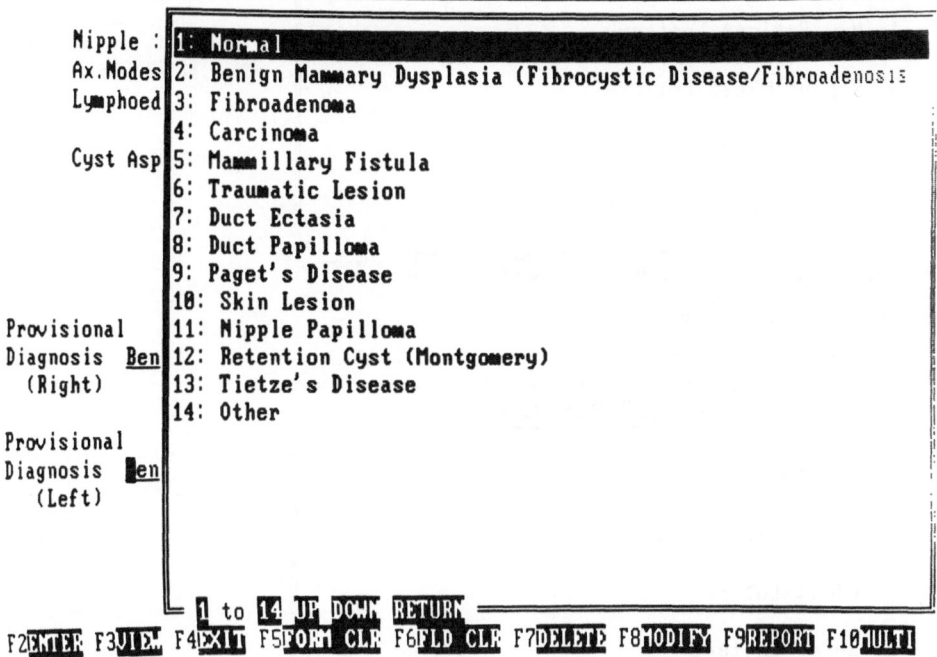

Fig. 1.5. New Patient Form showing the possible provisional diagnoses selectable from the on screen window.

histo pathologists, cytopathologists and radiologists are copied verbatim as free text to avoid potential misinterpretation.

At the end of every clinic the sheets and patient notes are collected by the secretary and the data transcribed from the sheets onto the forms in the database (Fig. 1.1). Entry into the database is password-protected and users can be defined as read, write, view or part-view only. At each stage the database is controlled by a series of predefined menus (Figs. 1.2, 1.3) and windows (Figs. 1.4, 1.5).

On completion of data entry, returning to the main menu permits alternative selections including letter and patient report printing, future clinic lists, and clinical audit. Printing letters (and reports) (Figs. 1.6, 1.7) is a date and patient name (wild characters e.g.* for all patients) dependent batch process (Fig. 1.8). Again a basic premise of the database structure relates to out-patient letters. The assumption made is that any given letter written about a patient will fall in to one of four types:

1. Admit
2. Discharge
3. Review
4. Refer

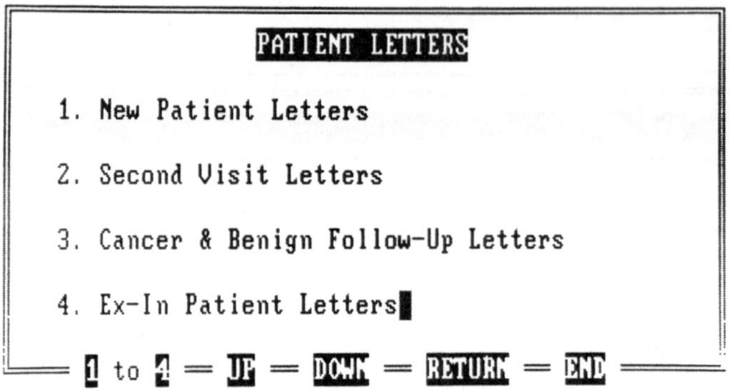

```
┌─────────────────────────────────────────────────────────┐
│                   ▌PATIENT LETTERS▐                       │
│                                                           │
│     1. New Patient Letters                                │
│                                                           │
│     2. Second Visit Letters                               │
│                                                           │
│     3. Cancer & Benign Follow-Up Letters                  │
│                                                           │
│     4. Ex-In Patient Letters█                             │
└──── ▌1▐ to ▌4▐ ── ▌UP▐ ── ▌DOWN▐ ── ▌RETURN▐ ── ▌END▐ ───┘
```

Fig. 1.6.   Patient Letter menu.

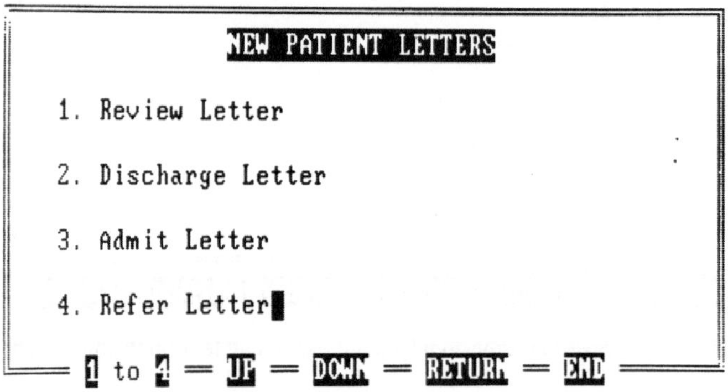

```
┌─────────────────────────────────────────────────────────┐
│                  ▌NEW PATIENT LETTERS▐                    │
│                                                           │
│     1. Review Letter                                      │
│                                                           │
│     2. Discharge Letter                                   │
│                                                           │
│     3. Admit Letter                                       │
│                                                           │
│     4. Refer Letter█                                      │
└──── ▌1▐ to ▌4▐ ── ▌UP▐ ── ▌DOWN▐ ── ▌RETURN▐ ── ▌END▐ ───┘
```

Fig. 1.7.   Menu of letter type selectable from New Patient Letters menu.

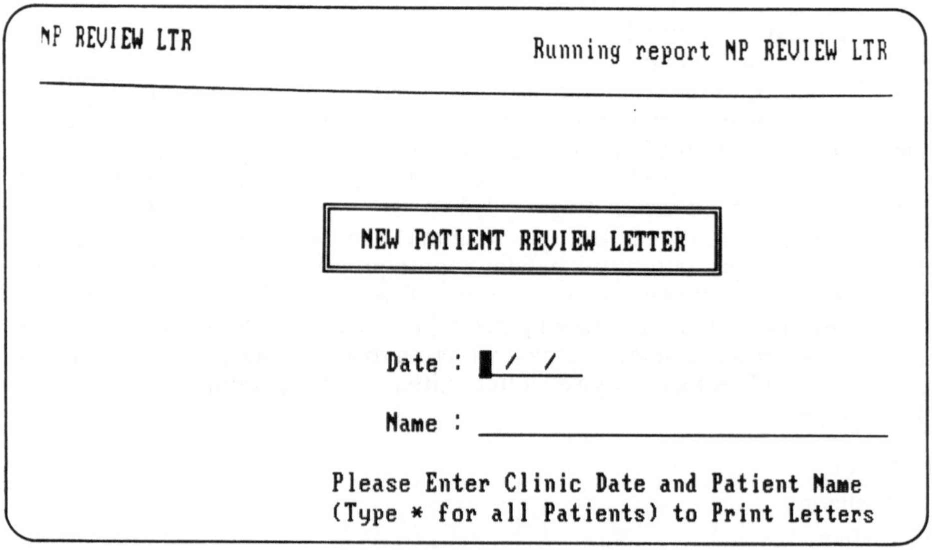

```
╭───────────────────────────────────────────────────────────╮
│  NP REVIEW LTR                   Running report NP REVIEW LTR
│  ─────────────────────────────────────────────────────────
│
│
│               ┌─────────────────────────────────┐
│               │    NEW PATIENT REVIEW LETTER     │
│               └─────────────────────────────────┘
│
│
│                   Date : █ /  /
│
│                   Name : _____
│
│               Please Enter Clinic Date and Patient Name
│               (Type * for all Patients) to Print Letters
╰───────────────────────────────────────────────────────────╯
```

Fig. 1.8.   Print menu permitting letter printing by date and patient name.

For each of the five patient categories already listed a separate standardised letter has been designed. For each of these 20 letters personal and medical data are abstracted from the database including the patient's and GP name and address, when the patient was seen, the diagnosis made, treatment proposed (or discharge) and new appointment or admission date given. These data fill the gaps (predefined fields) in the standard letters with the signatory being the doctor who saw the patient. Additional comments that the doctor wishes to make are automatically added as postscripts. These letters are printed on 3 part NCR (no carbon required (preprinted department-headed letter paper on an Epson EX 800 in NLQ (near-letter quality) mode at 120 cps (characters per second). Copies are then sent in window envelopes to the GP and/or referral source and a copy is retained for the clinic and hospital notes.

Printing of patient letters and reports is a batchable process which can be started and stopped at any place within the database. However, multi-tasking (i.e. printing and patient data input at the same time) is not possible.

Audit Capabilities

Basic clinical audit can be obtained through menu selection and gives attendance figures by patient category, numbers of patients seen by each physician, and surgical procedures undertaken and any complications encountered. The period of analysis can be specified by the operator. These and any additional ad hoc enquiries involve the use of the fourth generation programming language contained within DataEase. Complex record selection and comparison criteria, relationships, statistical analysis and report generation can be created. For example, listing, counting and giving the mean age plus standard deviation of all women who presented with a history of a breast lump who subsequently had normal mammography would be a relatively simple request.

The System in Use

Since 1 January 1987, 1456 women have been referred to the Bloomsbury Breast Clinic and entered onto the database. Patients who had already attended the clinic have not been included. Of these new referrals 816 were required to attend for a second visit, while 220 were ex in-patients, 260 have become benign follow-up and 78 cancer follow-up patients. This is equivalent to 5 971 223 Mbytes of data.

A total of 4 months elapsed from acquisition of the hardware and software to the present state of a fully functioning information management system. Subsequent modifications and improvements have been relatively minor and simple to implement. As the name of the software implies this information management has been relatively simple to set up, with no prior programming knowledge required. This represents a considerable advantage over the better known, but considerably less user friendly dBase III plus (Ashton–Tate), whose programming language is probably unnecessarily complex for this basically simple task. Clinically-relevant patient-related data have few of the complex relational and analytical requirements found in commercial databases.

Certain disadvantages to the approach employed for this management system have become apparent and are common in any database. First, having defined a field it becomes rigid – although it may be altered or re-defined at any time, data loss is a potential risk. For example, a field with several choice options cannot also have an option for text entry. Second, the chance for transcription errors is ever-present when data are transferred by a different person from the one who acquired the information. Third, technical support, ranging from the dealer to the software designer, needs to be easily on hand as system crashes (which to date have not occurred) can lead to significant work backlogs and disruption of the clinic.

In terms of cost this system has proved relatively inexpensive. With hardware costs of £3000, software costs of £400 and ongoing NCR headed paper printing of £130 per 2000 sheets. By avoiding professional systems developer costs (£250/day), considerable savings were made.

Conclusions

For computerisation in medicine to succeed various criteria need to be fulfilled:

1. Improvement over current systems
2. Acceptability
3. Feasibility
4. Upgradability

That this particular information management system continues to function efficiently nearly a year after its inception is a clear indication of its effectiveness and acceptability to secretarial staff and doctors alike. It must, however, be stated that computerisation has not meant a complete dispensing with normal clinic practices. The secretary continues to keep an admission and new appointments diary and does use her typewriter for long-term follow-up patient letters.

Our local GPs and oncological colleagues have been gratifyingly enthusiastic with the correspondence they receive from the clinic despite the necessary standardisation of letters. Whether such a system has a place in other out-patient clinics remains to be assessed.

Future enhancements include the customisation of a document reader to have the information from the sheets completed by the doctor entered directly onto the database without the need for keyboard entry. It is also hoped to develop an interactive expert system on a multi-user network which would propose management options derived from a rule-based knowledge system during patient interview.

Summary

Whilst the incidence of breast cancer remains relatively static the combination of an increased public awareness and the Forrest report on breast screening has placed increasing demands on NHS breast services. The limited range of breast disease management options coupled with the need for accurate record handling and analysis makes computerisation logical. Since 1 January 1987 a fourth generation programming language, menu driven, relational database (DataEase, Sapphire Systems Ltd) has been in operation in the Bloomsbury Breast Clinic running on a Tandon PCA 20 (20 Mbyte hard disc IBM AT compatible). Using a proforma identical to the on-screen forms (New Patient, Second Visit, Ex In-Patient, Benign Follow-Up, and Cancer Follow-Up) field data options are completed by the doctor examining the patient. As well as clinical findings, management recommendations (Admit, Discharge, Investigate, Refer) are selected on the forms. After the clinic these data are entered into the database and a report of the patient's visit plus a personalised letter to the GP/referring physician are printed (batch or individually) on hospital letter-headed NCR paper, copies being retained for the clinic's own files as well as being included in the patient's hospital notes.

Clinical audit capabilities include time period specifiable attendance diagnoses, discharge, admission and operation figures, as well as ad hoc comparisons. Full standard database functions such as record indexing, searching, scrolling and editing are also available.

To date, 1475 new patients (5.9 Mbytes) have been referred to the clinic and their first and subsequent attendances entered on the database. The implementation and the ongoing function of this information management system has met with a high degree of acceptability by the doctors, secretary, nursing staff and GPs. The design and use of database as a method of handling the routine information generated by a busy breast clinic has proved a practical and superior alternative to standard out-patient methods. Such systems may have wider uses in other clinics. Further proposed refinements include direct document reader data transfer and expert system development.

Acknowledgements. Grateful thanks go to Ms. Jill Bevan, Secretary to The Bloomsbury Breast Clinic whose industry and enthusiasm turned a concept into reality. The considerable contribution of both Mr. NB Sheikh and Mr. Adrian Cohen, Senior Surgical Registrar, is also gratefully acknowledged.

References

Haagenson CD (1971) Disease of the Breast, 2nd edn. WB Saunders and Co, Philadelphia, p 102

Nicols S, Waters WE, Wheeler MJ (1980) Management of female breast disease by Southampton general practitioners. Br Med J 281: 1450–1453

Pike MC, Henderson BE, Krailo MD, Duke A, Raj S (1983) Breast cancer in young women and the use of oral contraceptives: Possible modifying effect of formulation and age at use. Lancet II 926–929

2 A Microcomputer Multi-User Relational Database in a Department of Cardiology

I.C. Cooper, C. Carey, A. Crowther and M.M. Webb-Peploe

Introduction

While the traditional filing cabinet has proven value for the storage of data, it has significant disadvantages for information retrieval and analysis. Recent advances in microcomputer technology provide an alternative to the conventional approach. When considering this, it appears that there are a number of functions in a cardiology department such as ours which are particularly suited to computerisation.

1. The clinical work of three consultant physicians generates clinic letters and discharge summaries.

2. The department provides a service of diagnostic cardiac investigations (such as exercise electrocardiography, echocardiography and cardiac catheterisation) to other hospital departments and to other hospitals within the region.

3. The department is responsible for the administration of waiting lists for admission for cardiac catheterisation.

4. We are being increasingly required to provide an annual audit of the departmental workload.

5. There are a number of on-going research projects which depend on the ability to identify specific groups of patients and to retrieve information about them.

As there are increasing demands on our services we considered the introduction of a computerised database management system as a more efficient means of data handling with a view to improving the quality of service which we provide and reducing the workload on our secretaries.

Requirements

Before considering a choice of application we felt it was important to define precisely what the requirements of the system should be, and to adhere to these as closely as possible.

1. The application should allow multi-user access to all functions of the department, so that information may be shared between different users on a network.

2. The application should be user-friendly and those without any keyboard skills should be required to perform only the minimum of typing. The computer should be seen to be an easier alternative method of performing a particular task. For example, a secretary with no experience of word processing, should, with the minimum of training, prefer to use the computer rather than a typewriter to write a letter.

3. Data stored by the application should be updated as reports are generated and there should be no additional work involved in entering data simply to update the database.

4. The application should be written and maintained by us. We had found commercially available software for reporting cardiological investigations too inflexible to suit our specific requirements, and came to the conclusion that ideally those who would be using the application should be closely involved in its development. This has the advantage of independence of outside software support from the outset, so that modifications can be made to the system as requirements change in the future.

Description of the System

Software

We describe a relational database created using Omnis 3 Plus (Blythe Software, Saxmundham, Suffolk) running on the Apple Macintosh microcomputer. Omnis 3 Plus is available in both single and multi-user (up to 64 users) versions and is formatted for use with a number of different hard disc server and file server systems. It allows data files up to a maximum of 160 Mbytes in size, and each data file may consist of up to 24 related files. At present Omnis 3 Plus is one of the leading database management systems available for the Macintosh, both in the UK and in the US. Creating an application using Omnis 3 Plus is very similar in many ways to the procedure in other databases. However, there are important differences which we have found particularly valuable. The basic procedure is summarised as follows.

Creation of File Formats

The file format contains details of each field, including its name, type, length, and index status. In a relational database, such as this, a number of files are created and appropriate links between them are defined. An example of such a link would be between a file containing a list of patient details (file A) and one containing the results of a particular type of investigation (file B). Since each patient may theoretically have any number of such investigations, the link between file A and file B is described as a "many to one" connection. In other words file A has become a "parent" file to file B.

Creation of Entry Layouts

An entry layout is the computer screen design through which data are entered and displayed from the database. Within the entry layout a number of so-called temporary fields may be defined allowing calculations to be performed on the data (removing the need to store the results of the calculations). A powerful tool of Omnis 3 Plus is its own programming language with which short "sequences" or macros may be written. This allows the entry layout to be customised closely to particular requirements and, by programming "screen buttons" (rectangles on the screen, activated by clicking the mouse) and "pull-down menus", the screen will resemble the familiar Macintosh format.

Creation of Report Formats

Once file formats and entry layouts have been created, reports may be generated by the database. Report formats may take the form of lists or summary of information from several records in the database, or a report generated from single records from related files.

Creation of Menus

Access to an application may be organised by a system of pull-down menus. These are separate from the pull-down menus that drive sequences within the entry layouts, and provide a final link between the components of the application.

Creation of Passwords

Finally, if security is important, a system of multiple level passwords may be used to restrict access to certain files, entry layouts or report formats.

Hardware

Omnis 3 Plus runs on the Apple Macintosh microcomputer. We have used the Macintosh Plus which has a Motorola 32-bit 68000 processor, 1 Mbyte of RAM and a single 800 kbyte internal floppy disc drive. It is well known for its "WIMP" (Windows, Icons, Mouse and Pull-down menus) user interface. Macintosh Plus workstations are linked by the Appletalk Network and the number of terminals on such a network is limited only by the software (which allows up to 64 users). A number of Winchester discs and disc and file servers are available and the choice depends on storage requirements. We have used a 160 Mbyte hard disc and disc server (Symbiotic, Bracknell, Berks); 160 Mbytes being the maximum size of an Omnis 3 Plus data file. Printers include the Apple Imagewriter II (9 pin dot-matrix) and the Apple Laserwriter (300 dpi laser printer)

The Application

The first stage in the development of this application was the creation of a database consisting of two linked files (patient and exercise test files). The addition of new files allowed us to extend the application in a modular manner. At present the application consists of eight related files.

1. Patient file
2. Doctor file
3. Out-patient letter file
4. Exercise test and myocardial perfusion scan file
5. Echocardiograph file
6. Ambulatory electrocardiograph file
7. Pulmonary function test file
8. Appointments file

The file connections are summarised in Fig. 2.1. Each file is represented by a large rectangle, and each record by a line within the rectangle. In this example, a patient has a number of investigations, an appointment, a clinic letter (with a link to the referring doctor) and a general practitioner.

Patient File

This consists of patient details including name, date of birth, hospital number, address and telephone number. Since this file is connected to all files that require this information in the generation of their reports, an individual patient's details need only be entered on his first visit. In practice, when entering the results of an investigation, the patient's name is entered and an attempt is made to find that patient on the file. If the patient is already on the file the operator is able to proceed directly to entering the results of the test, whereas, if the patient cannot be located, the operator is asked to enter the details of the "new" patient.

Doctor File

Details of referring doctors are recorded only when a clinic letter is written and a patient is linked to the referring doctor via the connections formed with the letter file. The referring doctor may, of course, not be the patient's own general

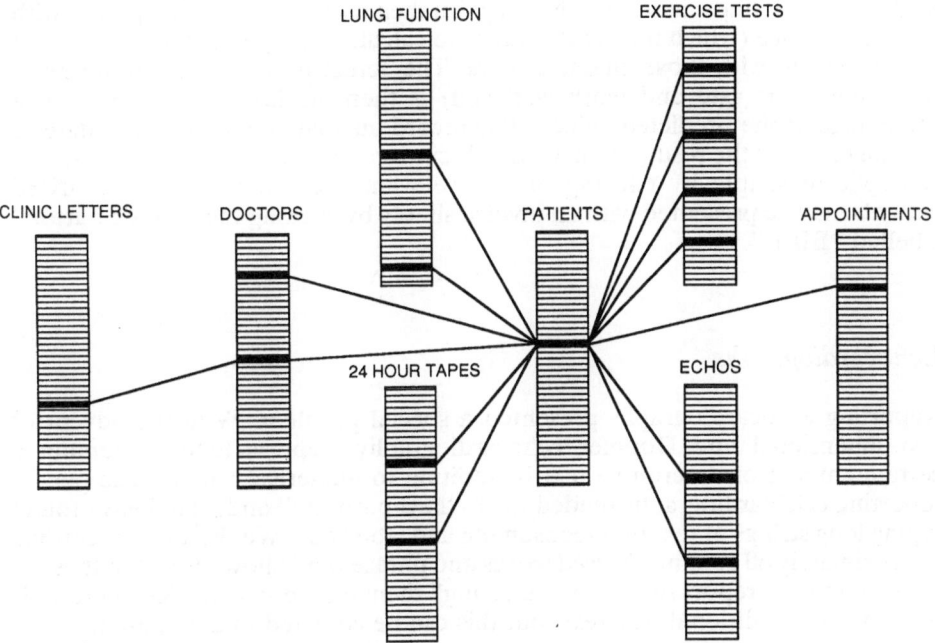

Fig. 2.1.   A relational database: files and file connections.

practitioner. However, since there is a one-to-many connection from patients to doctors, a patient may be linked to a number of doctors, one of whom is his general practitioner.

Out-patient Letters

A clinic letter is recorded for each patient and on subsequent visits to the out-patient department the previous letter is overwritten with a new one. The letter, which may be printed on a dot-matrix or laser printed, is formatted from details from the patient file, the referring doctor file and the letter file itself. This includes special fields for date of clinic visit, diagnoses and current medication. The letter may be structured with a series of section headings, or may simply be free text. The ability to enter free text is achieved by allocating one field per line and taking advantage of the word-wrapping facility between fields. Since many of our letters contain detailed reports of investigations, these may be included by selecting the relevant tests and "pasting" them into the letter, whence they can be subsequently edited.

Exercise Tests and Myocardial Perfusion Scans

The results of exercise electrocardiography are entered while the patient is on the treadmill. The operator is prompted to provide details of the patient's height, weight, activity status and sex. The program then uses these values together with the patient's age (which it has calculated) to calculate the performance expected of a fit person with those characteristics. The actual performance (in terms of maximum heart rate and work achieved) is then displayed, together with a percentage of the predicted values. The record may be edited at a later date to add the report of the results of myocardial scintigraphy. The report is then printed in duplicate simply by clicking on the relevant "screen button". Non-NHS patients may be presented with an invoice simply by clicking the "screen button" labelled "BILL".

Echocardiographs

Reporting echocardiographs presented a special problem. With the advent of two-dimensional and Doppler echocardiography, reports tend to contain a certain amount of descriptive text in addition to numerical values. The person reporting echocardiographs tended to be "keyboard shy" and would have found typing long strings of text time-consuming and laborious. We therefore identified approximately 60 commonly used words and phrases and allowed each of these to be included in a report simply by "selecting" them on the screen. The operator is able to enter additional free text, but this can be confined to a minimum.

Ambulatory Electrocardiographs

These are straight-forward brief text reports and present no special difficulties.

Pulmonary Function Tests

The results of spirometry are entered and the program calculates the expected values for the patient. If the results are abnormal, the report will provide an interpretation in terms of a particular ventilatory defect.

Appointments

This file holds records of appointments for myocardial perfusion scans. Appointments are displayed and spaces can be allocated to a new patient. A letter containing details of the appointment is generated if required.

Access to the files is achieved by a number of entry layouts each of which may be selected by using customised pull-down menus. There are individual entry layouts for each of the investigation files, clinic letters and appointments. Where appropriate, each entry layout will contain fields from other linked files. So, for example, the exercise test entry layout will contain fields from both the patient and exercise test files, hence forming a connection between a record from each.

Data may be entered or retrieved by using the entry layout for a particular investigation. This would be the method used by the technician performing the test, and may be used by others who require results. There is an alternative approach for those interested in the results of tests rather than in entering data. That is by an entry layout which is accessed by selecting "RESULTS" from the main menu. In this case the dates of all investigations for a patient are displayed. Data entry is not permitted in "RESULTS". Any of the tests may be selected and the results either viewed on the screen, printed, or "copied" for "pasting" into a letter. There is an additional option which automatically selects only the latest test from each category for that patient. "RESULTS" is therefore the most efficient way of retrieving results from different files and may be safely used by anyone without the danger of inadvertently inserting or deleting data.

The Network

We have used the Appletalk network. The Macintosh has a built-in networking capability within the ROM and the only additional hardware required are the cables to link the computers together. The system of cables and plugs are easy to assemble and we have been able to add computers to the network with no difficulty. Figure 2.2 shows the network in our department at present. It consists of seven Macintosh Plus computers, a 160 Mbyte hard disc and server, a 20-Mbyte hard disc (currently used for back-up), two dot-matrix printers and one laser printer.

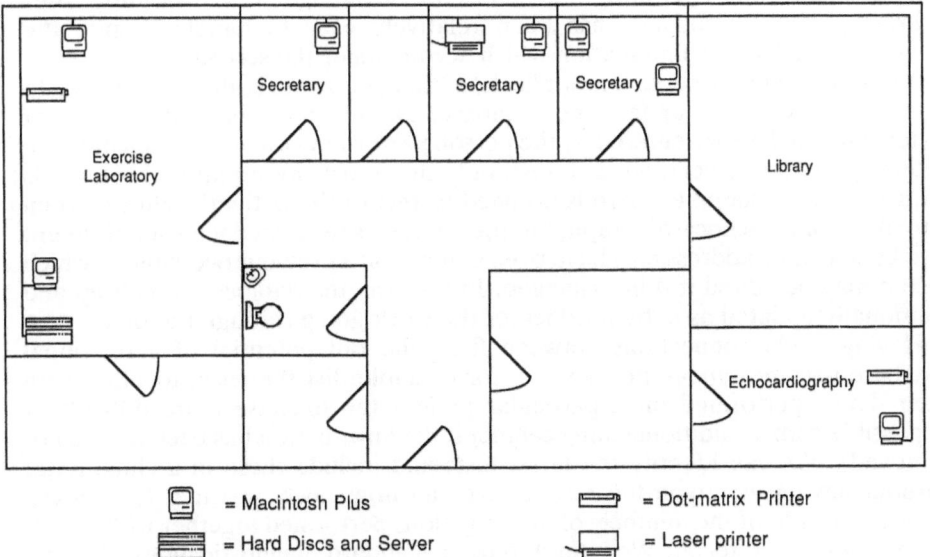

Fig. 2.2. Plan of department showing microcomputer network.

Discussion

We have presented the application in its present state of evolution. Clearly there are further aspects of the departmental work which are yet to be incorporated into the system. Initially we began by running the application as a two-file database for reporting exercise tests. This has since developed into a more complicated eight-file system and serves many functions. The fact that such a system can be created step-by-step (or file-by-file) is a clear demonstration of how it may be used to adapt to varying future requirements.

While the data management of our unit has similarities with that of others (thus making this approach relevant to them), there are certain unique aspects. Using a programmable relational database we have been able to customise an application to our specific requirements. For example, our application has built into it the exercise test protocol we commonly use. Unless software consultants are employed at great expense, no "off-the-peg" commercially available product would ever be able to achieve this level of detail.

It has been relatively easy to teach colleagues and staff to use the system. The secretarial staff (many of whom have had no training in word processing) have been very quick and eager to learn. The fact that this application has proved to be "user-friendly" is largely due to the fact that it conforms to the standard Macintosh format. The format, taking advantage of the WIMP user interface, is said to allow use of the computer to be intuitive rather than having to be learnt. It is also said that anyone with experience of using Macintosh software will find it easy to use new applications in the same format. This is not only true of the application we have created, but, perhaps more importantly, is true of Omnis 3 Plus itself. While one of the authors has some experience of programming in BASIC, none had previous experience of an application such as this. Programming an application in Omnis 3 Plus takes full advantage of the Macintosh user interface, and its language has been relatively easy to handle despite the frequently unclear documentation which accompanies the software.

It is important to note, in this application, that at no time is anyone required to enter data merely to update the database. Data entry occurs at the site of collection and data are entered by the person performing the test. When data are entered in order to generate a report, only the information required for this is requested. For example, there is no need to record the patient's address when attending for an echocardiograph, but the address is requested if an appointment is to be sent. The address may have been entered on a previous occasion, in which case it may be edited if it has changed. In this way the database is built up and continually updated as a 'by-product' of the work going through the unit.

Having made connections between files, the full potential of a relational database becomes apparent. We can, for example, list the tests, together with their dates, performed on a particular patient (an exercise more difficult or impossible with a traditional filing cabinet if the information has been misfiled or removed). We can identify the latest tests and include these in a clinic letter without having to retype the results. We can now easily provide, for a given period, an audit of the numbers of investigations performed together with details of the source of referral. We intend to use a standard diagnostic index so that a search can be made for certain groups of patients.

We have had some problems with the system. The networking of microcomputers and the use of a multi-user database such as this is still relatively uncommon in this kind of environment. A number of compatible hard discs, with different capacities, are available to serve an Appletalk network. We decided, from the outset, to obtain a large capacity disc in order to accommodate our needs for the foreseeable future. Unfortunately, it was only after catastrophic damage to the data file had occurred that it was realised that the disc server provided with the hard disc had allowed Omnis data to be inadvertently corrupted. In practice this meant that the use of the system had to be restricted only to those who could be relied upon to be diligently careful about the use of the computer. At the time (late 1986) this was the only disc server available to handle volumes of the size we had anticipated. It is only now (late 1987), that we believe a file server is available that will fulfil our requirements and the potential of Omnis 3 Plus. While it may be true that in general the technology already exists it seems that we have to be patient while manufacturers succeed in applying it to the realms of microcomputing. The software, however, has lived up to expectations and the few problems that have occurred have been minor.

It is impossible to make objective comparisons, but there is no doubt that this system improves our quality of output with legibily printed forms replacing handwritten reports. Most would agree (although proof is lacking) that producing a report or letter is easier on the computer than with the previous method. Our overworked secretaries understandably find it preferable to type only those parts of a letter that have changed since the last letter. Certainly the system has been acceptable to most people using it and it clearly has major advantages when it comes to retrieving results. The secretary does not have to leave her desk or use the telephone to find the result of any investigation performed in the department. Indeed it takes a few seconds to find the results of all the latest tests on a patient.

If one accepts that the local area network has a role in this setting, then a commercially available database management system such as that described would appear to be a powerful software option. We have seen how this product may be written and customised by those who will be using the system, and that prior knowledge of computer programming is unnecessary. Now that reliable hardware is available to support a system designed along these lines, this kind of application may have an important future in medical data management.

3 A Microcomputer System for Waiting-List Management and Audit

M.A. Walker, D. Bryce, J.L. Shearer and N.W. Carter

Introduction

The size of in-patient waiting lists has long been a source of concern to the public and to those working in the National Health Service (NHS). Recent NHS audit has demonstrated that some areas in the country continue to show an increase in waiting lists while in others a reduction has only been obtained by mailing those who have been on waiting lists for over three years. This has highlighted the need for more accurate audit and enquiry of existing waiting lists. In England a data set based on the Korner review was introduced in 1987. In Scotland the Information Services Division (ISD), recognising that the present waiting-list returns are inadequate, has developed a data set which is appropriate to Scottish needs. This new quarterly return, implemented on 1 January 1988, will, however, increase the workload of the already overburdened secretarial staff presently working in the NHS.

It is hoped eventually to base waiting-list management and hence the quarterly statistics around the Patient Administration Systems (PAS) which have been imminent for so long. It is our view that there may well be a place for a microcomputer-based waiting-list system at least in the short to medium-term until these PAS systems are installed. Furthermore, it is unlikely that every hospital in the country will have access to a PAS system hence the microcomputer option may well prove a long-term option to many of the smaller hospitals. Our objective was to create a microcomputer-based waiting-list management system to ease the workload of the secretariat and to provide an automatic facility which would produce, as a by-product, the new Scottish Home and Health Department (SHHD) returns.

The System

Method of Operation

The waiting-list system – known as CRAFTLIST – has evolved from CRAFT (Clinical Retrieval Analysis and Follow-up Template) which has been developed within our department (Walker, Bryce and Carter 1986) over the past few years. Indeed the major features of CRAFT were ideal for this application. The system is operated by a series of simple menus: the main menu is displayed below (Fig. 3.1). The first system, introduced in a urology unit, is operated solely by secretarial staff. Individuals are admitted to the computer system from waiting-list cards completed by the clinician in the out-patient department. Registration involves entering most of the demographic and disease data. When a patient is to be called, the relevant admission data are entered and those belonging to one consultant and for admission during a particular week are generated into a subset. Patients can be sent for singly although normal practice is to send for one week's admissions for each consultant in a batch. Once each consultant's subset has been generated using the management routines, the administration module permits the operator automatically to send personalised letters to each patient within each of the subsets. Patient ward lists and filing room lists can also be created for each consultant.

A routine also exists to generate a theatre list, basic information being obtained from the database. If a patient is cancelled or does not attend then this information is entered into the cancellation section of that individual's data file.

```
        WAITING  LIST   MENU




    1.    Admin letters


    2.    Enter Information


    3.    Data Management


    4.    Monthly Audit


    5.    Check Waiting List



Choose    1/ 2/ 3/ 4/ 5/ (H)elp/ e(x)it
```

Fig. 3.1.   Master waiting list menu.

Patients who have been admitted and discharged are either flagged as inactive waiting-list cases or given a date for repeat admission: those requiring further admission have a new disease dataset record appended to their file which then contains disease and operation data relating to their next admission. This method results in a chronological sequence of waiting-list and/or admission events which for a bladder tumour may extend over many years. Every month an audit is carried out, an automatic operation run overnight. This audit produces the appropriate figures for the new SHHD return. Ad hoc enquiries or analysis can be implemented at any time though a fuller understanding of the system is required to operate these facilities. We have also developed an extra facility to gather returns from a group of waiting-list systems to produce a single report by consultant, unit, speciality, and district or combination thereof.

The Waiting-List Database

The information contained within the database has been divided into three sections, demographic, disease and admission/cancellation data, as shown in Table 3.1. Although the example database has been generated for the urology department clearly it can easily be altered to cater for any other surgical speciality. Furthermore, the system could also be used for the management of an out-patient department. The operation and disease codes have been taken from the successful and well proven Coding System for Surgical Operations developed in the Lothian Health Board by the Surgical Audit Committee (1986).

Waiting-List Modules

Data Input

Each type of input transaction – for, instance registration, discharge or repeat admission – requires a different set of questions to be answered. In order to accommodate this efficiently an input form is generated for each of the recognised transaction pathways, each form only prompting answers to relevant questions. The forms presently held within the system – they may be altered at any time by the operator – are:

1. Registration
2. Repeat admission
3. Remove for waiting list
4. Cancellation
5. Admission data

Waiting-List Checker

This is a rapid look-up and check facility using either the individual's waiting-list number or name identifier. A simple surname and forename combination has been used as an identifier as patients seldom know their hospital number.

Table 3.1   Waiting-list data set

Demographic Information
    Waiting list number
    Surname
    Forename
    CHI
    Address
    Unique Identifier (Surname-Forename)
    Tel Number
    Sex
    GP Name
    GP Address
    Consultant
    Source Refer
    Min Notice
    Date put on waiting list
    Urgency
    Check flags

Recurrent Disease and Operation Date
    Disease Code
    Proposed operation
    Type of admission (D/C, GA, N/W)
    X-Rays and Hospital X-rays filed
    Comments (Social Constraints etc)
    Repeat admission/deferred admission/check cysto etc/child (check flags urology)
    Date to come in (if given at clinic)
    Actual op code
    Status waiting-list removal
    Date removed

Admission and Cancel Data
    Actual day TCI
    Ward to attend
    Time to come in
    Comments
    Type cancellation
    Reason if known
    Date of cancel

Administration Module

This important section of the system provides facilities to reduce secretarial workload by automating the regular weekly operations performed when sending for patients. Admission data are entered for each individual and the individual then becomes one of that consultant's subset of patients due for admission the following week. Once each consultant subset has been created it can be used to produce the appropriate personalised letter for one of the ten possible admission letters that have been set up for the urology department. The subset is then used to generate ward admission lists and lists for the filing room (Fig. 3.2) and X-ray department. It is also possible to create theatre lists through this module.

```
                    FILING   ROOM   LIST


        TUES    17      2301090069          JONES      Peter
                        30 Bridgend Street, Broughty Ferry, Dundee
                        Mr. Baxby          TUES 17           6  DRI


        TUES    17      240420183           SMYTH      Roger
                        49 Craigie Avenue, Dundee DD4 8LZ
                        Mr. Baxby          TUES 17           6  DRI


        TUES    17      1707110025          BLOGS      Grace
                        8 Kennet Road, DD3 6NS
                        Mr. Baxby          TUES 17           6  DRI


        TUES    17      1201460107          ANYONE     David
                        264A Hill Street, Dundee
                        Mr. Baxby          TUES 17           5  DRI


        TUES    17      1611360010          TOLLS      Robert
                        4 Gray Street, Monifieth
                        Mr. Baxby          TUES 17           6  DRI


        WED     18      1612040107          SMITH      Derek
                        13 Regent Road, Dundee
                        Mr. Baxby          WED 18            5  DRI


        FRI     20      1106750023          GOOD       Robert
                        19 High Street, Broughty Ferry, Dundee
                        Mr. Baxby          FRI 20            5  DRI


        FRI     20      0812470124          SMITH      Margaret
                        12 Backmuir Street, Dundee
                        Mr. Baxby          FRI 20            6  DRI
```

Fig. 3.2. Filing room list.

File Management Routines

Comprehensive data enquiry, analysis and manipulation facilities are included as an integral part of the software. Although many of the facilities are used in everyday operation of the waiting list the full potential of the options will only be utilised by someone with a good knowledge of the enquiry and analytical routines contained in the system. These routines provide for ad hoc enquiries or specialist and periodic analysis.

Much of the power of the system is provided by the ability to generate subsets from any item held within the database (Fig. 3.3). These subsets can then act as populations on which to perform both numerical analyses and non-numerical

```
   SUBJECT    CONDITIONAL    SUBSETS



   .1.   All on list                    2.   Remove 2832/1/87
    3.   All on list 28/2/87            4.   Males
    5.   Females                        6.   Mr. Baxby pat
    7.   Mr. Townell pat                8.   Mr. Weaver pat
    9.   D/C                           10.   IP
   11.   D/C to stay                   12.   IP + DC to stay
   13.   Check cysto                   14.   DC - check cysto
   15.   Mr. B IP M                    16.   Mr. B IP F
   17.   Mr. T IP M                    18.   Mr. T IP F
   19.   Mr. W IP M                    20.   Mr. W IP F
   21.   Mr. B's Adms wk beg. 22/3/87  22.   Mr. T's Adms for wk beg. Sun
   23.   Mr. T's Adms wk beg. Sun      24.   Mr. T's Adms wk beg. Sun 22nd
   25.   Mr. W's Adms wk beg. Sun 22nd 26.   Mr. B's Ward 23 D/C's Wed. 23rd
   27.   KB Adms 16/3/87               28.   PW 16/2 18
   29.   Remove 12/86-2/87             30.   Not made
   31.   NT ADMS 18/3/87               32.   Not made


   Choose which condition
```

Fig. 3.3.   Screen display of saved subsets.

tabular presentations (Fig. 3.4). Similarly reports or letters can be generated for each of those within a particular subset.

In summary these management utilities contain an integrated and sophisticated suite of routines which provide the operator with powerful and flexible tools to carry out extensive data enquiry and/or analysis on all data items held within the database without recourse to further programming.

Monthly Audit

At present the urology unit is required to produce a monthly audit of all those on the waiting list. The audit is split by consultant, day-case/in-patient, repeat admission, sex and waiting-list time. The automatic audit program has been created to perform the whole monthly audit as one task. The program produces one- and two-dimensional tables (Fig. 3.5) from which the appropriate figures can be extracted and placed in the form required by hospital management and ISD.

Auditing Several Waiting Lists

Each consultant's quarterly audit from a number of specialty waiting lists can be transferred into a further CRAFT data base. Each consultant is labelled by the unit, specialty, district and health board under which the waiting list is filed. This

1304 data points from a sample of 1304 subjects.
Sample is from a population of 1305 selected from **ALL** subjects.

KEY for X axis

Field 18 in File W/list:gen - Consultant
A = Mr Baxby
B = Mr Townell
C = Mr Weaver

KEY for Y axis

Field 13 in File W/list:gen - Sex
1 =   Male
2 =   Female

		?	A	B	C	TOTAL
?	N	6	1	1	0	8
	%R	75.0	12.5	12.5	0.0	
	%C	66.7	0.2	0.8	0.0	1%T
1	N	3	336	81	500	920
	%R	0.3	36.5	8.8	54.3	
	%C	33.3	71.5	64.3	71.5	71%T
2	N	0	133	44	199	376
	%R	0.0	35.4	11.7	52.9	
	%C	0.0	28.3	34.9	28.5	29%T
TOTAL		9	470	126	699	1304
	%T	0.7	36.0	9.7	53.6	

N = number   %T = % of Total
? = empty fields   %C = Number as % of Column total
                              %R = Number as % of Row total

Fig. 3.4.   Tabular analysis: sex v. consultant fields.

format permits audit of the figures by consultant, unit, specialty, district and health board in any combination as required (Fig. 3.6). In order to give the figures greater significance we have incorporated a facility to display the audit in terms of the last quarter, 6 monthly, 9 monthly or yearly intervals by any of the above combination of criteria (Fig. 3.7). This powerful and flexible audit tool will enable clinicians and administrators at health board or national level to monitor waiting-list trends. Note that Fig. 3.6 and Fig. 3.7 contain only data from a demonstration system.

November Audit In-patients

286 data points from a sample of 286 subjects
Sample is from a population of 939 selected from 6 subsets

KEY for X axis
Code and subset name
A = Mr W Male IP 133 5/12
B = Mr B Male IP 83 5/12
C = Mr T Male IP 8 5/12
D = Mr W Fem IP 24 5/12
E = Mr B Fem IP 38 5/12

KEY for Y axis
Field 20 in File w list:gen - Date put on W/L
1 = 1/80 to 11/83
2 = 12/83 to 11/84
3 = 12/84 to 11/85
4 = 12/85 to 5/86
5 = 6/86 to 8/86
6 = 9/86 to 11/86

		E	A	B	C	D	E	TOTAL
	N	0	22	13	7	3	9	54
E	%R	0.0	40.7	24.1	13.0	5.6	16.7	
	%C	0.0	16.5	15.7	87.5	12.5	23.7	19%T
	N	0	0	18	0	0	7	25
1	%R	0.0	0.0	72.0	0.0	0.0	28.0	
	%C	0.0	0.0	21.7	0.0	0.0	18.4	9%T
	N	0	8	12	0	0	8	28
2	%R	0.0	28.6	42.9	0.0	0.0	28.6	
	%C	0.0	6.0	14.5	0.0	0.0	21.1	10%T
	N	0	36	15	0	3	6	60
3	%R	0.0	60.0	25.0	0.0	5.0	10.0	
	%C	0.0	27.1	18.1	0.0	12.5	15.8	21%T
	N	0	31	12	0	9	3	55
4	%R	0.0	56.4	21.8	0.0	16.4	5.5	
	%C	0.0	23.3	14.5	0.0	37.5	7.9	19%T
	N	0	15	8	0	3	3	29
5	%R	0.0	51.7	27.6	0.0	10.3	10.3	
	%C	0.0	11.3	9.6	0.0	12.5	7.9	10%T
	N	0	21	5	1	6	2	35
6	%R	0.0	60.0	14.3	2.9	17.1	5.7	
	%C	0.0	15.8	6.0	12.5	25.0	5.3	12%T
TOTAL		0	133	83	8	24	38	286
	%T	0.0	46.5	29.0	2.8	8.4	13.3	

N = number   %T = % of Total
E = empty fields   %C = Number as N% of Column total
                                  %R = Number as N% OF Row total

Fig. 3.5. Tabular data presentation and analysis.

CONSULTANT		Male	Fem	Tadm	Radm	Def	In-P	DayC	DSty	Oadm	<3m	3-6m	7-12	13-24	25-36	>36m	TOT	Calld	Reavd
	Mr Pringle	226	140	300	80	9	300	60	6	0	45	78	120	80	34	3	374	34	36
	Mr Gunn	125	93	195	20	18	200	24	2	0	25	56	70	34	20	5	370	20	34
Unit 1		351	233	495	100	27	500	84	8	0	70	134	190	114	54	8	744	54	70
	Mr Davis	65	48	101	12	1	78	25	0	0	12	23	52	14	10	1	113	24	12
	Mr Peerce	167	120	260	20	7	245	35	7	0	24	48	76	53	24	2	288	34	23
Unit 2		232	168	361	32	8	323	60	7	0	36	71	128	67	34	3	401	58	35
Specialty -- Surgery total		583	401	856	132	35	823	144	15	0	106	205	318	181	88	11	1145	112	105
	Mr Baxby	220	138	165	120	12	218	114	4	0	30	78	96	60	40	20	365	70	45
Unit 1		220	138	165	120	12	218	114	4	0	30	78	96	60	40	20	365	70	45
Specialty -- ENT total		220	138	165	120	12	218	114	4	0	30	78	96	60	40	20	365	70	45
	Mr Walker	108	96	20	10	5	20	15	12	3	25	35	45	55	65	7	216	28	37
Unit 1		108	96	20	10	5	20	15	12	3	25	35	45	55	65	7	216	28	37
Specialty -- Opthamology total		108	96	20	10	5	20	15	12	3	25	35	45	55	65	7	216	28	37
	Mr Weaver	200	120	386	30	16	321	24	2	0	12	23	20	12	15	5	234	4	6
Unit 1		200	120	386	30	16	321	24	2	0	12	23	20	12	15	5	234	4	6
Specialty -- Urology total		200	120	386	30	16	321	24	2	0	12	23	20	12	15	5	234	4	6
	Mr.Lyall	950	20	100	47	25	98	67	201	34	279	305	46	59	34	48	1309	457	398
Unit 1		950	20	100	47	25	98	67	201	34	279	305	46	59	34	48	1309	457	398
Specialty -- Orthopaedics total		950	20	100	47	25	98	67	201	34	279	305	46	59	34	48	1309	457	398
Specialty -- Other total		0	0	0	0	0	0	0	0	0	0	0	0	0	0	0	0	0	0
DISTRICT -- DUNDEE total		2061	775	1527	339	93	1480	364	234	37	452	646	525	367	242	91	3269	671	591

Key

```
Male   =   Male
Fem    =   Female
Tadm   =   True admissions
Radm   =   Repeat admissions
In-P   =   In patients
DayC   =   Day cases
DSty   =   Day case to stay
Oadm   =   Other admissions
<3m, 3-6m, 7-12, 13-24, 25-36, >36m  =  Length time on waiting list
TOT    =   Total on waiting list
Calld  =   Total sent for
Remvd  =   Total removed from waiting list
```

Fig. 3.6. Quarterly waiting list returns, Dundee district.

Discussion

We have described a unit waiting-list management system which has been designed to be operated by secretarial staff. The development of a turnkey system based on CRAFT but with the added features required for waiting-list management has enabled us to provide an apparently dedicated system driven by a series of simple menus.

The choice of using stand-alone or networked IBM PC/AT compatible machines depends upon the local geographical and management requirements. One or more specialty lists may be run on one machine. We have developed an extra facility to gather returns from all such systems to produce a single report by consultant, unit, speciality and district, or by any combination of these parameters.

		Male	Fea	Tada	Rada	Def	In-P	DayC	DSty	Oada	<3a	3-6a	7-12	13-24	25-36	>36a	TOT	Calld	Reavd
Specialty -- Surgery	total	583	401	856	132	35	823	144	15	0	106	205	318	181	88	11	1145	112	105
		518	382	645	88	12	705	113	22	0	81	157	187	212	83	16	3475	88	70
		120	86	118	40	2	170	46	2	0	23	28	60	35	50	23	210	30	24
	9 mth total	1221	869	1619	260	49	1698	303	39	0	210	390	565	428	221	50	4830	230	199
Specialty -- ENT	total	220	138	165	120	12	218	114	4	0	30	78	96	60	40	20	365	70	45
		230	120	200	100	10	240	100	0	0	25	50	100	75	45	10	350	64	45
		0	0	0	0	0	0	0	0	0	0	0	0	0	0	0	0	0	0
	9 mth total	450	258	365	220	22	458	214	4	0	55	128	196	135	85	30	715	134	90
Specialty -- Opthamology	total	108	96	20	10	5	20	15	12	3	25	35	45	55	65	7	216	28	37
		0	0	0	0	0	0	0	0	0	0	0	0	0	0	0	0	0	0
		0	0	0	0	0	0	0	0	0	0	0	0	0	0	0	0	0	0
	9 mth total	108	96	20	10	5	20	15	12	3	25	35	45	55	65	7	216	28	37
Specialty -- Urology	total	200	120	386	30	16	321	24	2	0	12	23	20	12	15	5	234	4	6
		220	138	165	120	12	218	114	4	0	30	78	96	60	40	20	365	70	45
		0	0	0	0	0	0	0	0	0	0	0	0	0	0	0	0	0	0
	9 mth total	420	258	551	150	28	539	138	6	0	42	101	116	72	55	25	599	74	51
Specialty -- Orthopaedics	total	950	20	100	47	25	98	67	201	34	279	305	46	59	34	48	1309	457	398
		0	0	0	0	0	0	0	0	0	0	0	0	0	0	0	0	0	0
		0	0	0	0	0	0	0	0	0	0	0	0	0	0	0	0	0	0
	9 mth total	950	20	100	47	25	98	67	201	34	279	305	46	59	34	48	1309	457	398
Specialty -- Other	total	0	0	0	0	0	0	0	0	0	0	0	0	0	0	0	0	0	0
		0	0	0	0	0	0	0	0	0	0	0	0	0	0	0	0	0	0
		0	0	0	0	0	0	0	0	0	0	0	0	0	0	0	0	0	0
	9 mth total	0	0	0	0	0	0	0	0	0	0	0	0	0	0	0	0	0	0
DISTRICT -- DUNDEE	total	2061	775	1527	339	93	1480	364	234	37	452	646	525	367	242	91	3269	671	591
		968	640	1010	308	34	1163	327	26	0	136	285	383	347	168	46	4190	222	160
		120	86	118	40	2	170	46	2	0	23	28	60	35	50	23	210	30	24
	9 mth total	3149	1501	2655	687	129	2813	737	262	37	611	959	968	749	460	160	7669	923	775

Fig. 3.7. Nine monthly waiting list returns, Dundee district.

Examples have been drawn from the urology system which has now been operational for one year. A second, more ambitious, system which incorporates both in-patient and out-patient waiting lists has been operational in the orthopaedic department since the beginning of 1988. The simple tailoring required to accommodate other specialties involves configuring the new specialty waiting-list data files with the appropriate operation and disease codes, consultant names and special flags.

Looking to the immediate future we suggest that a small number of machines could easily maintain the waiting lists for a large hospital. It may be that each particular unit would wish to have its own system; however, if several units came under the umbrella of one system there would certainly be more cost-effective use of secretarial staff. Using this type of scenario the consultant would choose patients for the following week's admissions, using existing waiting-list cards or from an automatic waiting-list report produced by the system. This list would then be sent to the appropriate waiting-list operator who would maintain and run perhaps several "waiting-list units" and deal with enquiries by staff and patients. A "controller" would oversee each of the individual waiting-list units and would have a sound knowledge of the computer system thus enabling him to perform analysis and enquiry functions as requested by medical or management staff. Once each system was fully operational a monthly up-to-date catalogue of each consultant's waiting list could be produced in a predetermined format and sent to him, thus abolishing altogether the need for a card system.

The inclusion of the program to audit a number of individual systems gives clinicians and administrators alike the power to audit each system's data in a wider context without losing the advantages offered by the individual micro systems.

Looking further ahead, we are committed to eventual communication with the PAS systems. Our group has already exchanged data to and from our database with larger mini and mainframe systems. We therefore suggest that at the very least each of these individual systems could have their data downloaded into the PAS waiting-list module once fully implemented and the micro then used as a terminal to the mainframe system. If a suitable waiting-list module was not forthcoming then it would be possible for each of the waiting-list units to develop a symbiotic relationship with the PAS – indeed by using the microcomputer's processor rather than a "dumb" terminal it would be possible for the waiting-list system to utilise data held in the PAS system and also to update the PAS from information obtained from the day-to-day running of the waiting list.

Conclusion

We feel that this type of system is a very cost-effective way of achieving the required waiting-list statistics soon to be required by the Home and Health Department. The system also offers a more efficient way of managing unit waiting lists and leads to a reduction in secretarial workload.

References

Coding System for Surgical Operations (1986) Surgical Audit Committee Lothian. Roussel, Scotland
Walker MA, Bryce D, Carter NW (1986) A flexible clinical database. Br J Healthcare Comp 3: 15–17

4 Pacemaker Follow-Up System

K. Renner

Introduction

The Royal Sussex County Hospital is a large district general hospital serving a wide geographical area of East Sussex, and is the one accident and emergency hospital for the Brighton–Hove area. The district has an unusually high percentage of elderly people with the accompanying increased demand on medical facilities. The cardiac department manifests this increased demand in its pacemaker population.

Three and a half years ago, all details on pacemaker patients were held on card index file. Once a patient had been seen for a yearly or half-yearly check-up, the details were passed on to a departmental secretary who then typed a letter to the GP, informing him of the state of the patient. Because the secretaries had other duties, these letters were often delayed by a week or more. This was not the major headache. When pacemaker companies issued lists of pacemaker serial numbers which were suspected of early failure, the time and effort involved in trying to search out the respective patients was considerable. Different card index systems were tried in attempts to improve the system, but with little decrease in time and effort and with unreliable results. I was not convinced that when a pacemaker with a particular serial number could not be located, the patient was no longer under our care. Perhaps we had just mis-read the patient's card during the search.

I developed the present system when I was a physiological measurement technician, with no formal or informal computer training. My involvement with computers began when I agreed to key-in BASIC programs written by our consultant, Dr. Richard Vincent. From this I went on to write several respiratory systems in BASIC, and then began programming in dBase II and finally dBase III. The departmental technical and clerical staff now operate the eight different systems that I developed: I have returned to New Zealand but my role has been taken over by my fellow technicians. There are definite advantages in having the programs under one's control. It is easy to make enhancements or upgrades to the system, and the system exactly fits the requirements. It is not necessary to make do with a system that only approximates to requirements.

The First System

I began our computerised system on a BBC microcomputer, with twin floppy drives, which was already being used for simple word processing. The original assignment was to create a rudimentary list of all pacemaker patients to allow for easy recall. A simple file structure was created using BeeBase, and data on each patient were typed in. There were about 400 patients with pacemakers by this time, so we had to plan our alphabetical breaks carefully to fit in with the limited record capacity of Beebase. This caused some problems as it seemed that some alphabetical characters were more prone to cardiac electrical failure than others! However, we soon had a reliable search-and-find system working.

I continued with this system for some months, cursing the times I forgot to change from the A–E disc to the L–R disc when entering Peterson after Armstrong! The data soon spread over 5 floppy discs and a day and a half was spent on the computer for every half day in clinic checking patients and their pacemakers. An improved system was required!

The Improved System

Hardware and Software

An Apricot XI10 was purchased because of its portability, small footprint and large disc capacity – 10 Mbytes. Storage capacity has been increased by the addition of a Plus Five 20-Mbyte stand-alone unit with a 5-Mbyte removable cartridge system. This unit holds all back-up files, source code and a large research project. It has proven to be a reliable way to increase hard disc capacity.

Having spent numerous hours typing our pacemaker patient data into the BBC computer, I was rather anxious to avoid repeating the exercise. The Apricot is supplied with software which includes a communications package. This package was used to configure the Apricot as a printer. Patient data were transferred to the Apricot system by printing the BeeBase list to it. The data were now on the Apricot in ASCII text file structure. dBase II (Ashton-Tate, Oaklands, 1 Bath Road, Maidenhead, Berks SL6 4UH) has a useful facility which allows ASCII text files to be imported into the dBase format. I created a database file of a single field 30 characters long, to accommodate the longest field on the Beebase file. The ASCII file was read into that dBase file field by field using the syntax:

    append from <filename> delimited

A dBase II program was then written to read the simple file record by record and to place the data into the final format.

The facility to upgrade data from one computer to another and from one system to another is an important one. It is difficult to predict how large a system will grow, and how much disc space will be required, particularly when computers are used for the first time. With the exception of one system, all projects have grown larger and involved more data than anticipated. I have found that, with a little thought and manipulation, all data can be upgraded. This is obviously not desirable for every system but it is encouraging to know that projects can be undertaken without fear of size limitations.

Database Structure

I now had room to expand the record size, total number of records and additional facilities. For those unfamiliar with databases of this type, the file structure can be easily modified, shortened or lengthened depending on the whim and imagination of one's superiors! This is a feature of these products which makes them particularly user-friendly. The file structure has remained unaltered in the past 18 months or so, but previously was changed frequently. The programs were written in dBase II and compiled. The final file structure is as follows:

Patient Data Fields	Patient name
	Hospital number
	Date of birth
	3 address lines
	Phone number
	Name of GP
	Diagnosis
Pacemaker Information	Pacemaker and wire details
	Manufacturer
	Model
	Serial number
	Implant dates
Pacemaker Readings	Rate/P.W./Mag rate for
	Set readings
	First ever readings
	Latest readings

Date of Patient's Next Appointment

Using the Patient Database

The Patient Database has two indexes, the patient name and the hospital number. I thought that the hospital number could be used as a unique key, and entering that would always bring up the patient details. This has been found unsatisfactory in practice. While a hospital number is unique to each patient, one patient may have more than one hospital number, particularly if he has been to several of the hospitals in the area. To further compound this problem, our district has recently computerised on the PAS system, and in doing so has allocated new numbers to the patients. A patient with three different hospital numbers is now not an unusual occurrence. I have found in all the systems presently in use, that a more reliable key is the patient name. The operator may still search on the hospital number, if desired.

Using the Pacemaker Database

The Pacemaker Follow-up System is menu-controlled which makes it more user-friendly and requires less operator training. I found this to be an important consideration, particularly when the operator had little computer experience. There is also a certain amount of fear on the part of older people faced with a computer. Simple, fail-proof steps go a long way to overcoming that fear and engendering confidence in the operator. The system is called up from a batch file which selects the relevant subdirectory, starts the database and performs automatic back-up to the hard disc when the system is closed down.

The main menu (Fig. 4.1) appears after the unique user password has been entered. To get to this point the operator has to do the following:

1. Turn on the computer
2. Type in the name of batch file – in this case PACER – which has been displayed for him on the screen

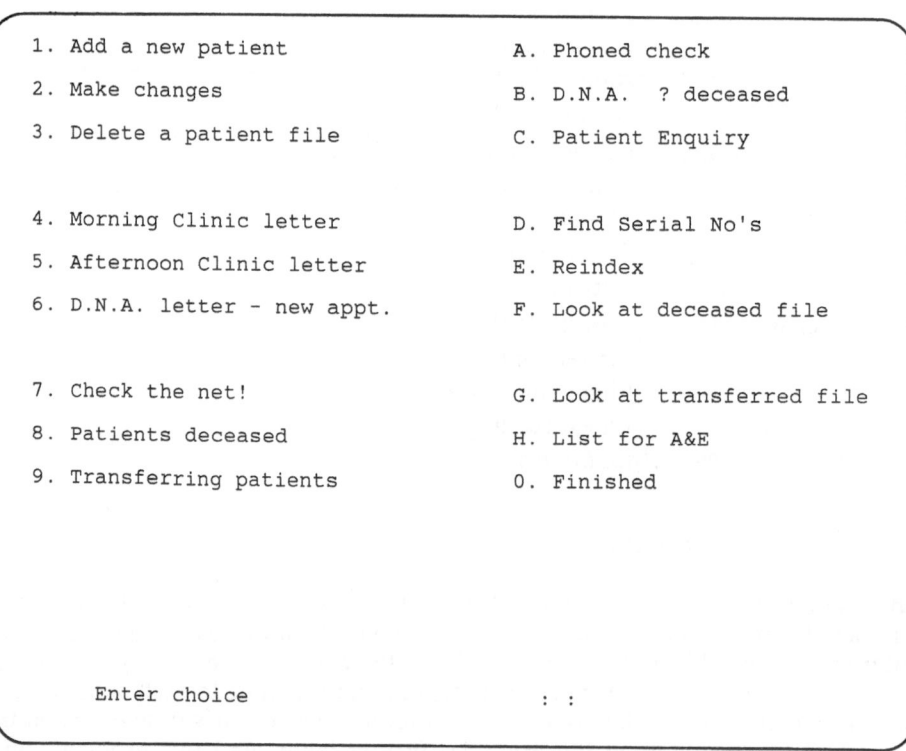

1. Add a new patient	A. Phoned check
2. Make changes	B. D.N.A. ? deceased
3. Delete a patient file	C. Patient Enquiry
4. Morning Clinic letter	D. Find Serial No's
5. Afternoon Clinic letter	E. Reindex
6. D.N.A. letter - new appt.	F. Look at deceased file
7. Check the net!	G. Look at transferred file
8. Patients deceased	H. List for A&E
9. Transferring patients	0. Finished
Enter choice	: :

Fig. 4.1. Main menu for the pacemaker system.

3. Enter his password (the only thing he has to remember)

4. Accept or alter the default date that is presented

5. Select the required option from the menu

The first three options on the main menu allow for the addition, alteration and deletion of patient details. These were the first programs to be written, but are now used infrequently.

A patient may be found by typing any abridgement of the surname. A list corresponding to those letters is printed on the screen with the patient record number, hospital number and date of birth displayed.

For example, on entering BRO the following patients might be displayed:

000189	BROACH JAMES	K893552	12/05/23
000335	BROADBENT MICHAEL	K220603	18/06/34
000698	BROWN ANGELA	K102054	05/11/12
000259	BROWN ARTHUR	K116953	29/03/05
000492	BROWN MARTIN	K120856	31/09/11

The operator has only to enter the corresponding record number and the patient details are displayed using the template shown in Fig. 4.2. This method of use forms the entry into almost all the programs in the suite. The advantage of this is two-fold. Firstly, the operator quickly learns the layout and is familiar with programs that are run infrequently. Secondly, the programming is much faster when a basic template is used from which to program.

Serial Number Check

The main priority – a register of patients conforming to pacemaker serial numbers – can be quickly and easily created from option D in the main menu. The serial number is entered into the computer which then checks through the serial number field in each record to try and match the string. Once found, the details are displayed on the screen. This process takes a very short time, even with a large database.

Missed Appointments

I also created a way to ensure patients did not miss appointments without our knowledge. This is of major importance, particularly with an elderly population of pacemaker patients with poor memories. Without a fail-safe method of checking that all patients have been seen at least once a year, appointments would be forgotten and pacemaker rates would fall to unsatisfactory levels. A program was written to ensure that no patient goes more than a year without a check-up. This program can be run at any time and prints details of all patients who have no follow-up date in the "next appointment" field. This list also includes patients whose follow-up date is before the current date. These patients can then be checked on and given new appointments where necessary.

```
                        Add a new patient


   Name              :                              :


   Hospital number:          :

   Date of birth   :  /  / :

   Address -1       :                             :

          -2       :                             :

          -3       :                 :  Phone :               :

   G.P.             :                         Diagnosis   :                :


   P.M.manufact.   :    :            Wire manufact. :                :

   Model           :            :    Model    •    :              :

   Serial number   :            :    Serial number :             :

   Implant date    :  /  / :         Implant date   :  /  / :


   Set rate    :  0:        P.W.   :0.00:      Magnet rate :   0:

   First rate  :  0:        P.W.   :0.00:      Magnet rate :   0:

   Programmable   : :


   Correct? Y/N    A TO ABORT      : :
```

Fig. 4.2. Capturing patient and pacemaker data.

Letter-Writing System

A large part of the system is devoted to creating letters. Early in the development of the system, the operator would select a letter option and search for a patient. If the patient had not yet been entered, the operator would have to return to the menu, select the option to add a new patient, add the details, return to the menu and then return to the letter option to print the letter. This was obviously time-consuming and frustrating. The system was altered to allow the operator to add new patients to the file from the letter option. If the patient is not on file, by selecting "A" to add the details, the Add Details program is called. Details are entered and the operator is returned to print the letter. Much effort was avoided by making the programs modular in this fashion.

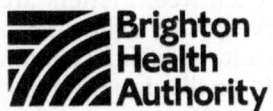

Cardiac Department
Royal Sussex County Hospital
Eastern Road
Brighton BN2 5BE
Tel· Brighton (0273) 696955
Please ask for extension 4211 /4214

Your ref

Our ref

                                                           11/12/87

Dear Dr Vet

              re: BEAR EDWARD (01/01/01) Q123456
                   1 Ashdown Forest, Sussex

     We saw this patient in our pacemaker clinic today
     and confirm that the system is working satisfactorily.
     The pacemaker rate is set at 70 pulses per minute.

     The heart-rate may be faster than this without suggesting
     any fault, but the rate should not fall below 65
     beats per minute.

          Only the electrical system was examined; if you
     feel there is any need for a cardiological opinion
     please let me know.

          Another pacemaker check has been arranged for
     12 months time.

                                      Yours sincerely,

                                      Mrs S.Baker
                                      Chief Cardiac Technician

Fig. 4.3. Typical letter to a GP after a pacemaker clinic.

At the end of the pacemaker clinics, which are held each week, letters are printed to the GP informing him of the patient's check-up, the state of the pacemaker, and our future follow-up plans (Fig. 4.3). The additional information needed to create that letter, above the patient details held on file, is very small. The technician has to enter the latest pacemaker readings into the computer when the patients are seen. The only details that must be added above this, for the letter to be printed, are the number of months to the patient's next appointment, the lowest allowable rate of the pacemaker, the initial of the doctor seeing the patient an the initial of the technician. There are two variations of this letter, a morning clinic letter when the patient is not seen by a doctor at the clinic, and an afternoon clinic letter for patients who have been seen by a doctor. Two copies of the letter are created – one for the GP and one for the patient notes. This saves secretarial time and avoids time delays between seeing the patient and informing the GP. The letter-writing system is summarised in Fig. 4.4.

In addition, letters are also created to inform a patient who failed to attend for a check-up when his new appointment has been set for. A letter can also be printed giving full details of a patient's pacemaker system when he is transferring to another hospital. This letter, although used infrequently, saves a lot of time and ensures that all the patient's details are sent to the new centre. The letter includes a checklist of other papers which may need to be enclosed, thus serving as a reminder for the technician.

Initially letters were printed on a dot-matrix printer, but the department has recently invested in an Epson laser page printer. This quickly produces excellent quality letters on hospital-headed paper.

Additional Facilities

We also keep databases for patients who have been transferred and for patients who have died. This allows us to keep better track of patients: a superior method to deleting them from our working file when they are transferred by the hand of God or man. Listings of these files are available at the press of a key. This has been a more recent development to the system, but one found to be invaluable.

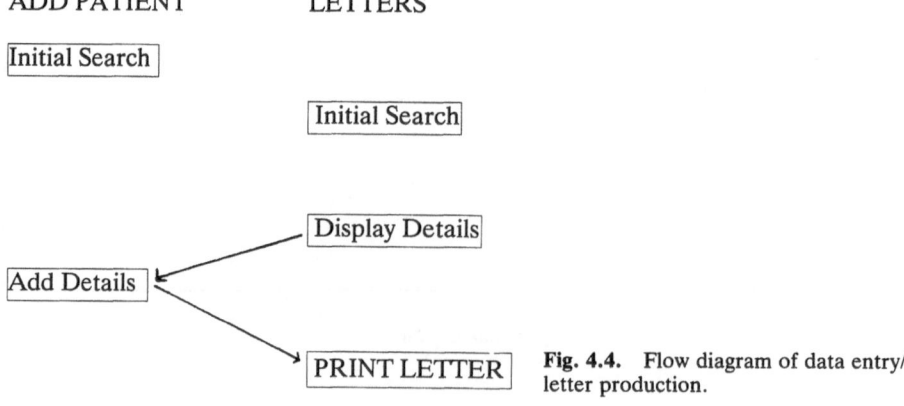

Fig. 4.4. Flow diagram of data entry/ letter production.

Instead of assuming a patient is dead or transferred because he is not on our working file, his status can now be verified and further investigation initiated if his record is not found.

Value of the System

The Apricot, on which this system operates, also runs four other applications. The financial outlay for the hardware in terms of the pacemaker system is therefore relatively small. The system has more than paid for itself in terms of both secretarial and senior technician time saved. The system requires no secretarial time at all. Although the technician must spend a small amount of time entering data after each pacemaker clinic, this is more than compensated by the ability of the system to provide useful information. Automation of repetitive tasks is economic from both a financial and a time perspective.

I am satisfied that the system now fulfils the requirements of its users. An afternoon clinic of 30–40 new patients can be added to the computer and letters created in a total time of 2 hours. Statistical data are available using dBase III in immediate mode. No time is lost in waiting for letters to by typed and no additional secretarial services are needed. The technician in charge of pacing has total control over the record keeping and has instant access to information. The system has proved reliable and has increased confidence that the follow-up of pacemaker patients is secure.

Address for enquiries regarding the system. Dr. Richard Vincent, Department of Cardiology, Royal Sussex County Hospital, Brighton BN2 5RE, UK.

Further Reading

Bodner MS (1986). Plan before you plunge. Data Based Advisor 4: 25–27
Computer Systems. Computer Users Guide and Handbook (1985) pp. 40–93
Desposito J (1987) File managers get a face lift. PC Magazine 6: 119–133
Poor A (1987) Database power puts on an easy interface. PC Magazine 6: 109–117

5 Development of a Microcomputer-Based Patient Administration System Using Omnis 3 Plus on the Macintosh

N. Watson

Introduction

Patient administration systems (PAS) have been, or are being, installed in many British hospitals. Unfortunately, there are no software or hardware standards, so that the day-to-day workings of these systems vary from region to region, and even from district to district within regions. This is a pity, to say the least. Furthermore it is the case that, in most hospitals, the terminals used to access the PAS are dumb, that is to say that they are merely screens with keyboards and possess neither memory nor computing power. Every task to be undertaken must be carried out using the software installed on the hospital mainframe or minicomputer. There are inevitable constraints and limitations in these circumstances. Only the software that forms part of the PAS is available. It is the case that any PAS is necessarily administration orientated. That is not surprising. That is its purpose. But doctors who both wish and need to have a more individualised administration system for their practice or department are continually frustrated by PAS. Quite simply the systems so far installed just do not, and cannot, provide what they would like. Even where audit programs have been added to PAS they remain rather inflexible.

The dramatic progress of the personal computer in the last 5 years, brought about by ever-increasing memory capability, means that it is now practically possible to develop software that will deliver a desk-top PAS suitable for an individual doctor. Using networking and multi-user software versions, groups of doctors may be served. These can, of course, be linked to bigger hospital systems. Commercially available relational databases have enabled enthusiastic doctors to develop such systems without any prior programming knowledge.

Database Design

Single files will not be sufficient to represent all medical data in a particular clinical practice. Files of patient details, a file of GP names and addresses, a file of diagnoses etc. can certainly be useful, but it is only when these files can be made to relate to one another that a useful database can be constructed. For example, entering a diagnostic code in a patient's file can be made to pull out that diagnosis in words when it comes to write a letter or report. The construction, and inner workings, of a medical database are likely to be complex but the front end (that part which the user sees) must be both easy to understand and intuitive in its workings. Minimal training should be required in order to use the system. In practice that is a tall order and means a lot of work.

Hardware and Software

Of the microcomputers available, the best known and most widely used in Britain are, almost certainly, those made by Amstrad, or by IBM, together with its clones. But, in my view, the software for these machines, and particularly the database software that is commercially available, is relatively difficult both to learn and to use. Indeed the machines are not altogether user-friendly. By contrast the Apple Macintosh works in a more intuitive way. Omnis 3 Plus, a commercially available relational database (Blyth Software, Milford House, Saxmundham, Suffolk) offers all that is necessary to produce turnkey solutions to specific data problems, with the added advantage of being able to produce an end-product which utilises all the advantages of the Macintosh operating environment. Having made a decision to use Omnis 3 Plus on an Apple Macintosh, together with a 20-Mbyte Hard Disc, design of the system began.

File Structure

Although readers of this book are likely to be familiar with common jargon used in describing and developing databases, one or two basic items require emphasis. The fundamentals of file structures are of great importance. What is meant by file structure? It is a question of deciding which (electronic) filing cabinets are going to store which (electronic) files, and which (electronic) documents are to be stored in which (electronic) files. More demandingly, it also means giving very careful consideration to the possible links that might exist between information stored in different documents, different files and different filing cabinets. This is the relational part.

In a simplistic way a good example would be to decide where GP names and addresses should be stored. Clearly they need not be on every patient record. The same name would appear in many records. The solution is to store a list separately, and recall the appropriate details by giving each GP a code number. In that way only the code number need be entered and stored in the patient details. Then decide where, in the other pieces of information, the GP's details will be required. Letters to GPs and discharge summaries would be obvious examples. Patient detail files must be linked to GP detail files, letter files and summary files to allow transfer of the appropriate information. It should by now be clear that the whole of a practice needs to be carefully analysed so that a database may be constructed in such a way as to produce a system which will store all the information required. The information must be readily and speedily accessible. Most importantly the information must be held in such a way that it can be amalgamated, or merged, to reduce repetitive, time-consuming and boring office tasks, in short to produce a hosptial doctor's office administration system, as opposed to a hospital administration system.

The Independent Practice, Administration and Retrieval System (IPARS)

The system now to be described is called IPARS, an aconrym of *I*ndependent *P*ractice, *A*dministration and *R*etrieval *S*ystem. This was a learning exercise and has taken 750 hours to develop. If you are to start from scratch with little or no computing experience, be prepared for a long haul. I suspect that a similar undertaking using dBaseIII on an IBM would probably have taken a lot longer. But only a powerful relational database will allow you to finish up with what I am describing. Use a simpler database by all means, but don't expect the degree of automation and complexity that the more elaborate programs provide. By and large you get what you pay for.

So, what can IPARS do, and what does it look like? It can:

Store patient details
Store Master Lists of
    GPs
    Referring consultants
    Solicitors and insurance companies
    Diagnoses
    Drugs
    Tests
    Procedures
    Complications
Record patient's diagnoses, drugs, tests, procedures and complications
Produce standard or individual letters
Automate discharge summaries
Maintain appointment lists and send appointment letters
Maintain operating lists
Maintain waiting lists
Provide searching facilities
Provide accounting facilities

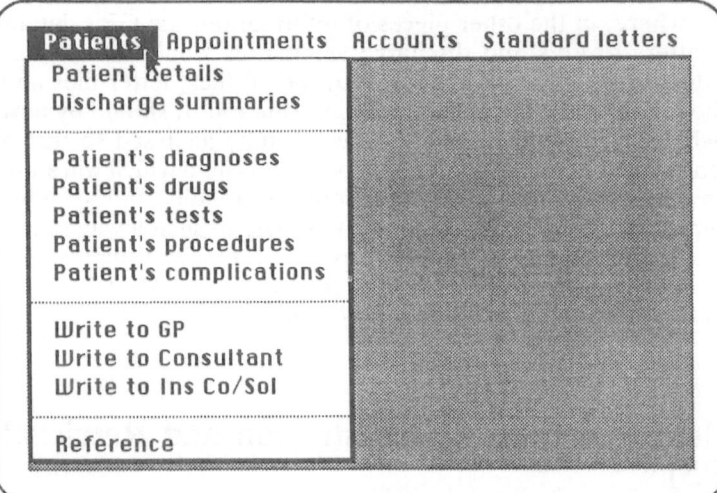

Fig. 5.1. On launching IPARS the Patients, Appointments, Accounts and Standard Letters menus appear after the normal apple, file and edit menus. The illustration shows the patient's menu pulled down.

What Does IPARS Look Like?

Figure 5.1 shows the appearance of the screen on start-up. The top line appears adjacent to the standard Apple, File and Edit menus. Pulling down the Patient's menu produces the items shown. At any one time an individual patient's list of diagnoses, or whatever, may be accessed from the same menu. Selecting Reference takes you behind the scenes, and three new menus replace the last three on the start-up screen. Pulling down the Reference menu (Fig. 5.2)

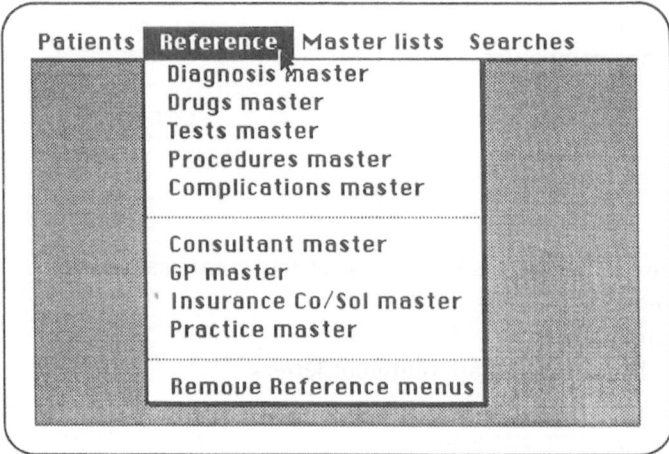

Fig. 5.2. The effect of activating Reference from the Patient's menu. 3 new menus appear. The Patient's menu is retained.

provides access to add to or modify the Master lists. Any one of those lists may be printed, either to the screen or to a printer by activating the appropriate section of the Master lists menu. The Searches menu requests entry of the necessary information required for simple searches.

Returning to the start-up menu provides the mechanism for day-to-day activities, which include correspondence, appointment and waiting-list management, accounts and standard letters. The standard letters have to be compiled for individual users, but the rest of the system is really suitable for most, if not all specialties, though individual tailoring will be necessary to deal with variations in office and practice procedures.

Data Entry

The workings of the entry screens have been designed to be as uniform as possible. Figure 5.3 shows the Patient Details screen. The fields for data entry are self explanatory. The entry date is entered automatically by the system. To be noted are the buttons present on the right-hand-side of the screen. Note that one is dimmed (change). That is because there is no current record to change. The single word commands are activated by a mouse click, so that there is no need to pull-down other menus for data entry, or to remember complex keyboard commands. In some sections a keyboard alternative to a mouse click is available. Once a patient's details have been entered IPARS allocates a number unique to that patient. On any subsequent occasion that the patient's details are required

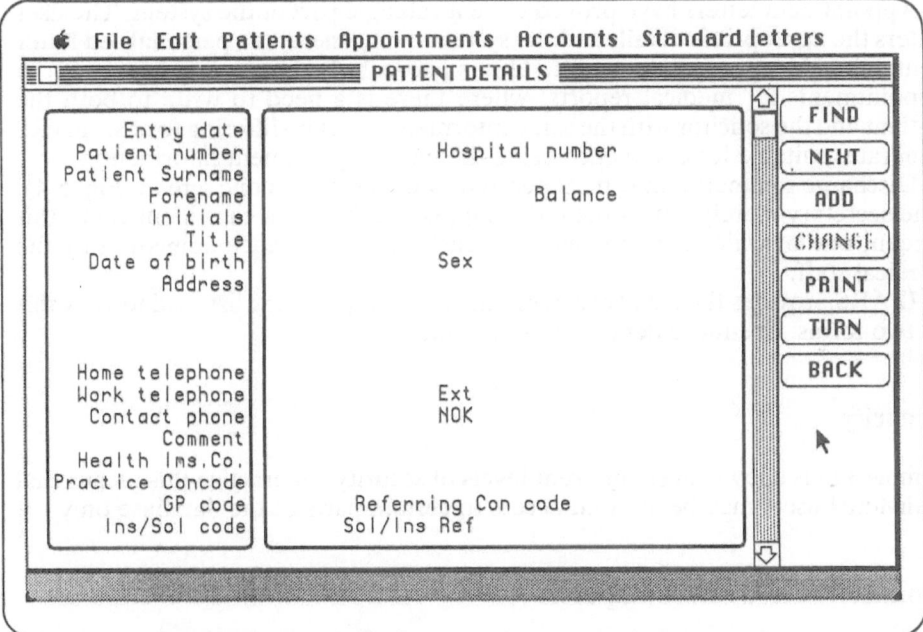

Fig. 5.3. The front sheet for entering patients.

simply entering that number will procure all the relevant details from the patient's file. "Balance" is a display-only field showing the current balance owed by the patient or insurance company, a figure derived from the integral accounting system.

In the Reference section separate entry screens are provided for all the Master files, and the Reference lists can be printed to screen or printer at any time.

The letter-writing facility is probably the work horse of the system, and a part likely to provide real savings in secretarial time. Data entry simply requires insertion of a patient's number. Text is then entered and the print command marries up the patient's details, the target for the letter (i.e. GP, another consultant, insurance company or solicitor) and finally adds the appropriate details at the foot of the letter. The word-processing facilities are simple, using standard Macintosh techniques, and the page actually consists of 42 linked text fields. The standard letter section has also been well received and much used in practice, particularly the DNA (did not attend) letters. Individual users will clearly require customisation of these letters to suit their own speciality and style of practice.

The accounting system is based on the idea of episodes. Every time a patient makes contact is an episode, i.e. consultation, operation, preparation of medical report etc. These episodes are then stored. When the time comes to send a bill the user selects those episodes to be billed. They may be PP (private patient), or MR (medical report) episodes. The command print then sets out the selected episodes in chronological order, totals them and enters the date and amount in a separate file used for sending reminders. Obviously PP episodes are billed to patients and MR episodes billed to insurance companies or solicitors, hence the need for two separate pathways.

Appointment letters have proved to be a valuable part of the system. The user enters the appropriate details and the system then generates a personalised letter containing the appropriate details. This is particularly time-saving in relation to appointments for medical reports, where there is a need to write to both the patient and the solicitor with the same information, but in differing forms. IPARS generates suitable letters to each using the basic appointment information.

Discharge summaries may be generated by data entry on one screen (Fig. 5.4). The secretary merely enters the data, supplied to her on a card identical to this screen, one of which is maintained for each patient for each admission by the medical staff.

IPARS provides the facility to maintain a desk-top waiting list, and to view this in two forms, one more detailed than the other.

Security

Omnis 3 Plus allows seven different levels of security. In practice this means that individual users may be allowed access to certain parts of the database only.

Connection to Other Computers

Although it is a simple matter to connect a Macintosh, and most other microcomputers, to hospital PAS systems, there are problems. The present state

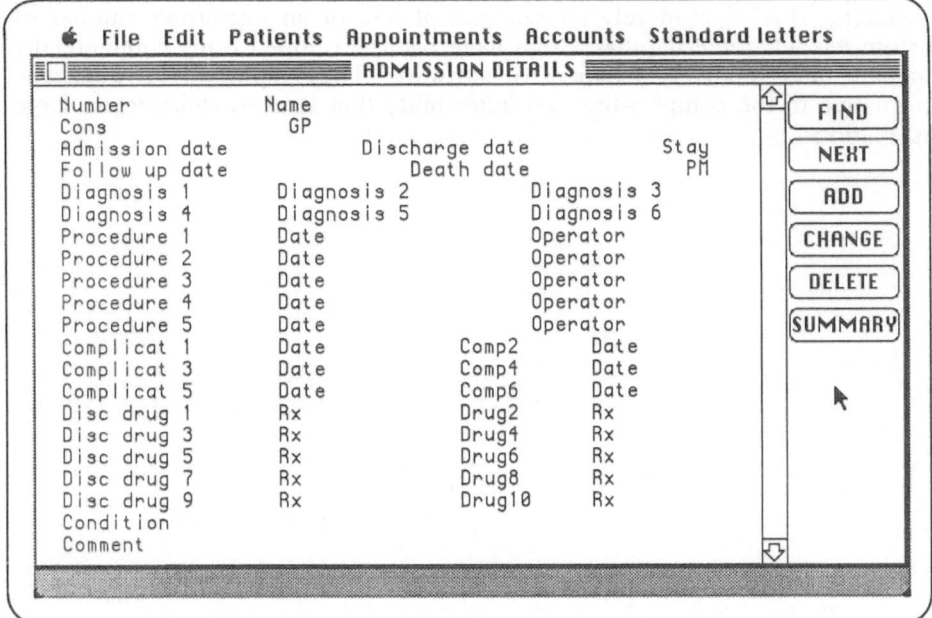

Fig. 5.4. The data entry screen for discharge summaries.

of development will enable the microcomputer to act as if it were a dumb terminal. This is easily achieved by installing the appropriate terminal emulation software in the microcomputer. I have found Mac 240 (Whitepine Software, 75 Route 101A, PO Box 1108, Amhurst, NH 03031, USA) to be excellent.

The problem, and the challenge, lies in the difficulties which currently face us in relation to the ability to upload or download information to or from the hospital computer to the desk-based micro. Simply grabbing a screenful of the hospital computer's information is easy. But unscrambling it and putting it into a desk-based database poses a number of problems which are beyond the scope of this article. In many hospitals, such data transfer is impossible. But there is every reason to be optimistic. Once data transfer has been achieved, the place for the customised desk-based relational database will really be established.

The Future

Mass storage techniques will greatly change microcomputer capabilities in the future. CD ROM will be the most important of these. CD stands for Compact Disc and ROM for Read Only Memory. About 100 000 pages of text can be stored on one CD and so with a CD player a microcomputer will be able to get at quantities of information which it has hitherto only been possible to store on very large installations. Indeed, the whole trend towards minis and micros is inevitable. IPARS is merely an example of one of an increasing number of customised relational databases that have been developed using commercially available and relatively inexpensive software. They represent an attractive alternative to the complexities and inflexibility that tend to characterise large installations.

6 Computerised Management of Intensive Care Unit Data

J.R. Colvin and G.N.C. Kenny

Introduction

Optimum management of the critically ill patient requires frequent monitoring of many variables and an ability to detect and act upon significant changes in patient condition at an early stage. This intensive monitoring leads to the rapid accumulation of vast amounts of data in which significant changes in patient condition may remain undetected (Osborne et al. 1968). This type of data collection is ideal for handling by computer, which allows clear presentation of informative and relevant aspects of the information. The improvement in data presentation should result in fewer management errors by the clinician (Jenkins et al. 1968), and in the early detection and correction of adverse trends (Kenny and Campbell 1982).

If a computer system is to be successfully implemented in a clinical environment it should fulfil the following criteria (Glaeser and Thomas 1975; Phillips, Gordon and Cousins 1982):

1. The output from the system must provide bedside information which is relevant, accurate, reliable, accessible and familiar
2. The output must be appropriate to local procedures
3. Data input must be simple, to prevent interruption of patient care routines and to improve accuracy of data collection
4. Retrieval of information must be simple, even for occasional users
5. The system will only work satisfactorily if introduced without staff opposition, and if the users believe that the system is of value to them and their patients

Therefore, in addition to careful selection and planning of the computer equipment necessary for a particular application, account must be taken of acceptability, ease of use, and user friendliness when designing specific software.

Initial computer applications in medicine required centralised mainframe or minicomputers with multiple peripheral terminals to provide the required speed and processing power necessary for handling the data. The drawback of these systems lies in their requirement for highly trained staff to program and operate them, and in their great cost. In addition, a fault in the single processing system results in loss of function of the entire system.

Rapid advances in microprocessor technology have led to the availability of powerful, relatively inexpensive microcomputers, which may be interfaced directly to the patient monitors, allowing frequent data collection and processing to a suitable display format such as a trend graph on the computer screen. Fluid balance figures or laboratory results can be entered manually or by the methods described below.

The power and versatility of microcomputers in intensive care can be further enhanced by a network system incorporating, in addition to individual patient bedside computers, a hard disc storage unit and additional computer linked to a printer. Networking allows common access to shared peripherals, with increased transmission speed and storage capacity. It removes the need for floppy disc storage with its high risk of disc contamination or damage and consequent loss of information. Such a system has been developed in the Respiratory Intensive Care Unit (RICU) of Glasgow Royal Infirmary, and is described below.

Description of System

Hardware

The system in use in the RICU is based on Apple IIe microcomputers and the Corvus Omninet (Corvus System Inc., 20290 Toole Ave, San Jose, California, USA) network. Each bedside Apple is provided with colour visual display unit (VDU) and is interfaced to the patient monitor via an Apple II Super Serial Card which is set to operate at 9600 baud. The monitors in current use are the Kone 565A (Gambro Ltd, 47 Leesons Hill, St. Mary Cray, Kent, UK) and the Roche 128 (Kontron Ltd., 52 Telford Road, Cumbernauld, Scotland) models.

The analogue arterial waveform produced from a transducer must be converted to digitised form by an analogue-to-digital converter (ADC) to allow processing by the computer. Some monitors (Kone 565A) have in-built conversion and their output of digitised information may be input directly to the computer. This connection must maintain electrical isolation between the monitor and computer to comply with electrical safety regulations. This can be achieved by the use of an optical coupling as described by Kenny and Davis in 1983. The Corvus Winchester hard disc has a 16-Mbyte capacity, and is situated in an undisturbed corner of the ward. In addition to the standard mains power supply it is provided with battery back-up from a Powerbank 500 uninterruptable power supply (Power Testing (UPS) Ltd., 23 Tallon Road, Brentwood, Essex).

Three further Apples are incorporated into the network. One, at the nurses' station, allows entry of fluid balance and laboratory results, and permits remote monitoring of one patient's cardiovascular information. A second, in the secretary's office, is connected to a dot-matrix printer which is used to produce a daily print-out of each patient's data and a hard copy of all stored information to

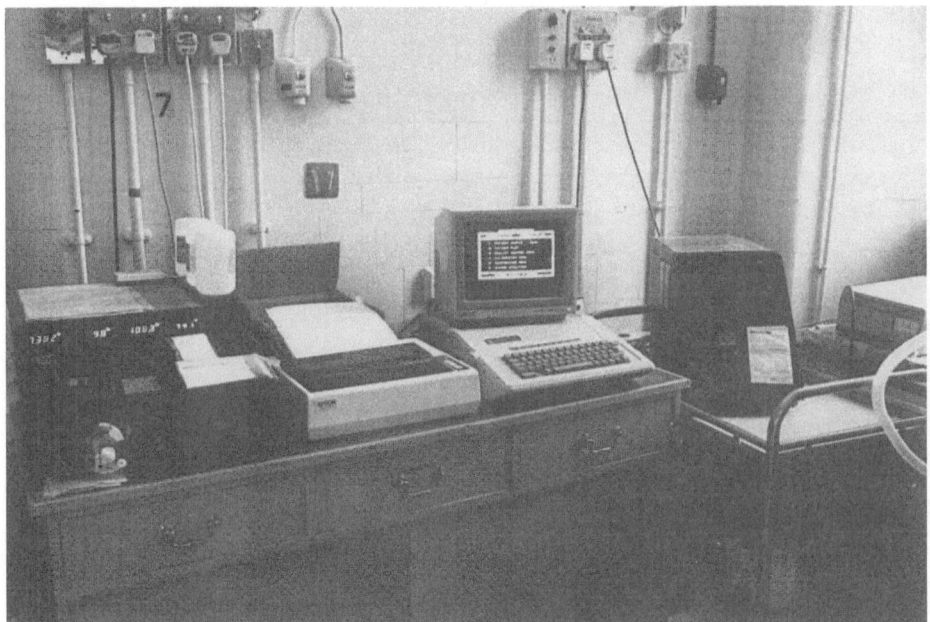

Fig. 6.1.   On-line data collection from blood gas analyser.

be transferred to the patient's case record on discharge. This computer may be used for entering laboratory results, and both these patient-remote systems are available to run the teaching programs and the proforma program for analysis of RICU statistics. Any program development can also be undertaken away from the patient environment. The third Apple is interfaced with a Corning 178 pH and blood gas analyser and with a second dot-matrix printer (Fig. 6.1). This provides on-line collection of blood gas results and automatic print-out of the new data together with the four previous results for that patient. Blood gas data are stored on-line and can be interleaved with cardiovascular data collected at the patient's bedside, for calculation of oxygen delivery and consumption.

The network connections are made by a simple twisted pair cable and allow transmission at 1.2 megabaud. The microcomputers communicate with the Corvus via a transporter card and are individually coded by setting the numbered dip switches. Each Apple is provided with a clock/calendar card with battery back-up using Thunderclock (Thunderware Inc., PO Box 13322, Oakland, California, 94661, USA) Mountain Hardware (Mountain Computers Inc., 300 Harvey West Boulevard, Santa Cruz, California, 95060, USA) or Proclock (Practical Peripherals, 31245 La Baya Drive, Westlake Village, California, 91362, USA) boards.

Software

The programs to operate the system are all stored on the Corvus hard disc, and may be loaded to each computer as necessary. Access to the files is safeguarded

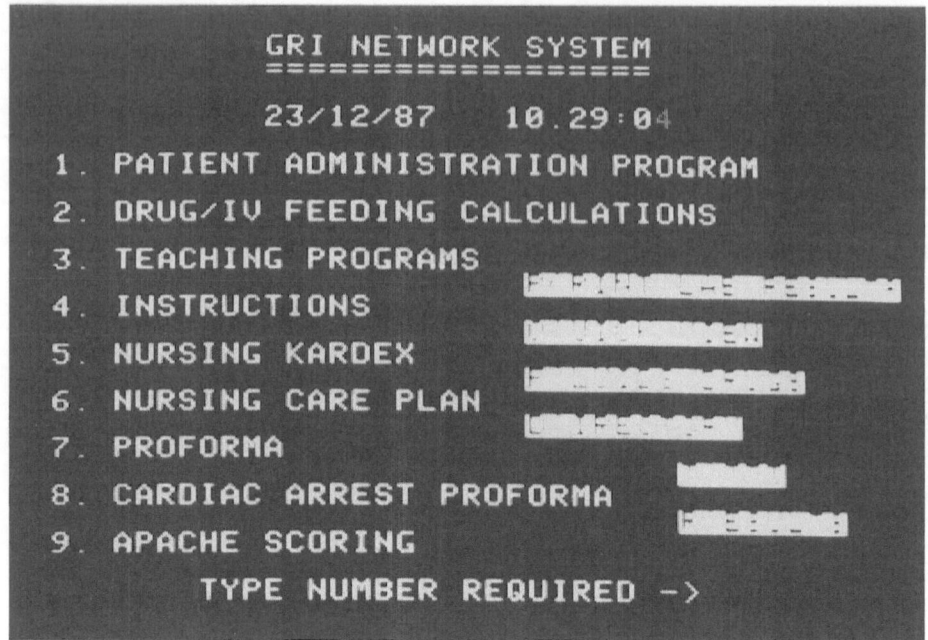

Fig. 6.2. Main menu screen of RICU network.

by inserting a password step in the start-up routine thus limiting the use of the system to authorised personnel only. The options available are presented as a series of numbered menus allowing easy selection with number and RETURN keys only. The main menu, permitting access to all the network's facilities, is shown in Fig. 6.2. In addition to patient data collection and processing programs, this allows access to the teaching programs, nursing care plan programs, and the general RICU and cardiac arrest proformata. The Corvus also stores a suite of system checking and maintenance programs to enable any faults to be rapidly diagnosed and corrected by the technical staff.

The full range of data processing options and facilities are discussed in more detail below and are conveniently subdivided into data collection, storage and utilisation.

Data Collection

Data may be saved automatically, by on-line collection, or entered manually by various methods. On-line data collection is appropriate for frequent saving of rapidly changing variables, including cardiovascular pressures and rate information. In addition to the electrical safety aspects discussed previously, several factors must be considered when planning an on-line collection system. The program must be able to detect and eliminate artefacts produced by blockage, damping or flushing of the arterial line. The input for the arterial pressure transducer must be correctly zeroed and calibrated; and the program must include the correct calibration factor for each computer/ADC/monitor combination. The system can store information as frequently as every minute, but is more commonly set for quarter-hourly collection. It is programmed to display the information as a trend graph on the colour VDU in addition to transmitting all the data to the patient's file in the Corvus hard disc. The system can be used to collect heart rate, systemic and pulmonary systolic, mean and diastolic pressures, central venous and capillary wedge pressures, and cardiac output. Core and peripheral temperatures may also be stored. If used with a suitable ventilator, such as the Sieman's Servo 900C (Sieman's Ltd., 28 Napier Court, Ward Park North, Cumbernauld, Scotland), respiratory information can be collected on-line, and processed by the computer to produce derived information such as compliance/resistance characteristics, and flow/volume loops (Davis, Kenny and Campbell 1982). This information can be used to identify optimal ventilation for the patient, and to assess effects of bronchodilators or other therapeutic manoeuvres.

The other area in which on-line data collection is in routine use in our RICU is for results of blood gas analysis. The results are automatically collected and paired with the appropriate patient information such as mode of ventilation and inspired oxygen concentration. They are transferred to the Corvus and printed as hard copy with the previous four blood gas results.

Many types of data are not suitable for automatic input to the computer, therefore off-line data collection is used to enter such information; for example, patient administration, fluid balance, laboratory results, drug doses, and to provide a facility for entry of free text comments. If it is to be accepted by clinical staff, the computer must appear to offer significant benefit over manual charting. Data entry, therefore, must be simple and non-tedious, with a minimum of keyboard work, and with error trapping routines to prevent the collection of invalid information. (The disadvantages of the standard 'QWERTY' keyboard include its vulnerability to damage in a clinical environment and the relative degree of skill necessary for its efficient operation.) With these aims in mind, the system in our unit makes use of numbered selection menus for access to each section and the use of simple YES/NO options where possible. A light pen can be used for many types of data entry and is cheaply and simply produced from a pen casing and photo-electric cell. It is easily used by the non-expert to enter data by touching the appropriate part of the screen (Fig. 6.3). However, the light pen may not function well in very brightly lit areas.

A recently installed ATARI ST system of bedside computers in the postoperative cardiac intensive care unit (CICU) utilises a "mouse" for users to communicate with the computer.

Data Storage

The main database program of the network system has the capacity to hold complete sets of files on 16 patients at any given time. This spare capacity, over and above the seven active patients who may be in RICU, allows some delay in removing files after discharge. This is important as the secretarial staff are not

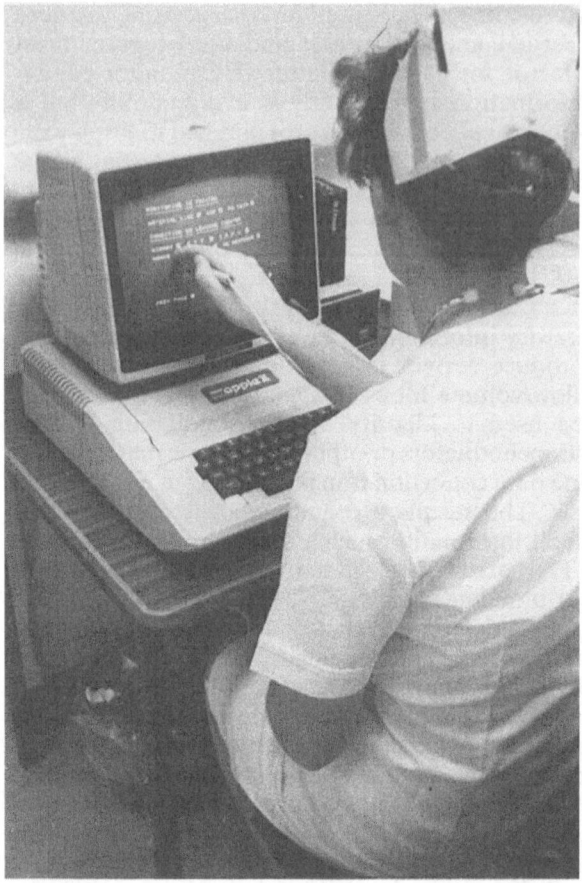

Fig. 6.3.   Use of the light-pen in RICU.

available to complete the discharge summaries of patients who have left the RICU out of hours. Each patient has a file opened on admission, which is indexed in the active file list under the patient's bed-space, name and hospital number. Any relevant results and clinical details are also entered at this time. The file is kept in this active capacity for the duration of the patient's stay, during which time information may be added or extracted as required. On discharge, the patient file is removed from the active list to an interim list of patients awaiting the preparation of discharge summaries. This patient summary, of code numbered boxes, is completed by the secretarial staff using stored information from the network. In addition a print-out of laboratory and clinical details is transferred to the patient's case notes. The bulk of the patient information is then deleted from the main data base, a limited amount being transferred to the RICU proforma file for statistical and audit purposes. In addition to patient identification data, this file stores information about referral source, progress and outcome of the patient's stay in intensive care, and about the nature of the pathology. A third, smaller, database is used to store details about cardiac arrests occurring throughout the hospital. This information is entered manually by the duty registrar using a light-pen and allows audit of the functioning of the "arrest team".

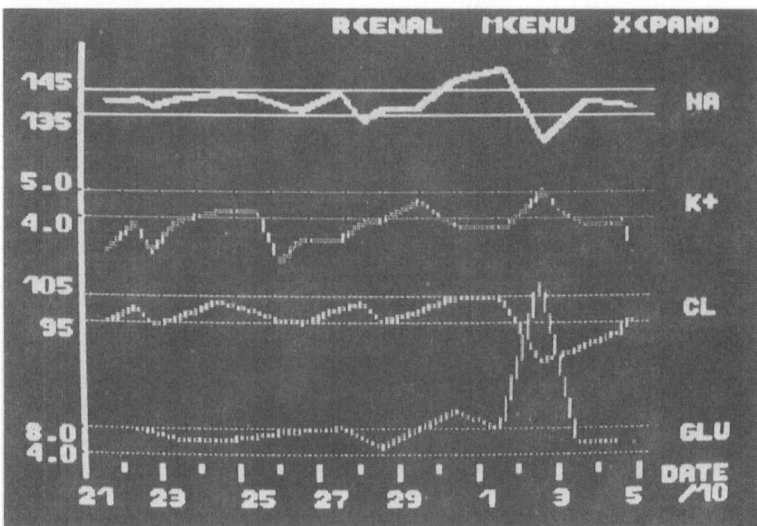

Fig. 6.4. Typical trend graph of serial results.

Utilisation of Data

The primary function of this system is to organise collection and presentation of the patient information in the most useful form. In addition, much use may be made of this information for direct and indirect patient care, for statistical analysis and audit, and for research purposes. Some applications, currently in use in our intensive care unit, are described below.

Direct Use

A variety of trend graphs can be displayed on the VDU by selection from a series of simple numbered menus. These can be set to varying time scales as desired. This function may be used to display cardiovascular trends, blood gas trends (with added derived respiratory data), and trends in various laboratory results. An example is shown in Fig. 6.4.

Information may also be displayed in tabular form, under individual patient indexing or under the heading of each variable. Thus electrolyte results, for example, may be viewed as either a particular patient's results over several days, or as a list of all the patients' electrolyte results for a particular day (Fig. 6.5).

Indirect Use

Specific software may be designed to use the basic data for derivation of indirect information. Examples in current use in our unit include calculation of intrapul-

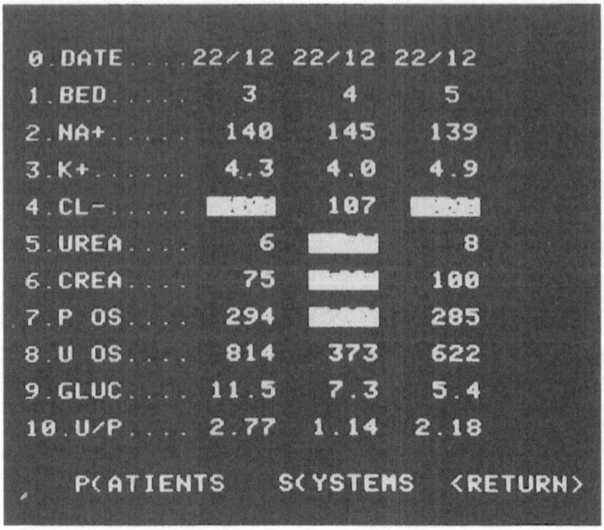

```
 0.DATE ....22/12  22/12  22/12
 1.BED.....    3       4       5
 2.NA+....   140     145     139
 3.K+......   4.3     4.0     4.9
 4.CL-.....          107
 5.UREA....    6               8
 6.CREA....   75             100
 7.P OS....  294             285
 8.U OS....  814     373     622
 9.GLUC.... 11.5     7.3     5.4
10.U/P....  2.77    1.14    2.18

   P<ATIENTS     S<YSTEMS    <RETURN>
```

Fig. 6.5. Tabular format of results presentation; abnormal values are highlighted.

monary shunt and derived cardiovascular variables, such as cardiac index, left ventricular stroke work index and oxygen delivery. Complex respiratory information may be derived from on-line ventilator data. A combination of multiple variables can be used to decrease the frequency of false activation of alarms (Stewart 1982). This program correlates several simultaneous variables and alarms only occur if a combination of events stray outside preset limits. Alarms can also be set to warn of specific abnormalities in individual waveforms, such as sudden blockage or disconnection of an arterial line, or spontaneous wedging of a pulmonary artery catheter.

Patient information is used to calculate the requirements for intravenous feeding. This program collects the necessary data from the patient's file and calculates the patient's fluid, calorie, protein and electrolyte requirements for the following day. After asking for input on any specifically contra-indicated feeding solutions, it then suggests a regime for the patient which may be printed and used to order the prescription from pharmacy. Another facility uses the patient's weight and manually entered information to calculate intravenous drug infusion rates required to deliver a specific drug dose. A recently introduced program calculates each patient's *Acute Physiology And Chronic Health Evaluation* (APACHE) score. Again, the information is taken directly from the patient file, or entered manually, and serial calculations may be obtained. Suitable data can also be used in closed loop therapy. The computer system in the CICU uses the input from direct arterial pressure and a manually entered target pressure to control the rate of infusion of vasodilators in postoperative cardiac surgical patients.

Research Uses

Computerised data collection offers a reliable and unbiased source of data for research. Examples include a current study of a new inotrope/vasodilator drug which requires recording the cardiovascular response to therapy over 48 hours and serial information on certain electrolyte and haematology variables. Another example is the collection of cardiovascular data in the evaluation of closed loop blood pressure control systems (Reid and Kenny 1987).

Statistical Analysis and Audit

The proforma program allows manipulation of information in the proforma data base to provide statistics about the RICU since 1983. This includes monthly figures, overall mortality numbers and information on referral sources and the numbers of various types of pathology admitted.

Conclusion

The aim of installing a networked microcomputer system was to make optimum use of the information available, and to reduce the time spent on paperwork by clinical staff. The use of on-line data collection and computer-based records in intensive therapy units has been shown to increase nursing time spent on direct care from 2% to 24% (Sheppard 1979), and to reduce time spent on clerical duties from 19% to 7% (Miller, et al. 1978). In addition, this system will continue to function during acute crises and periods of clinical stress when the nursing and medical staff are fully occupied, and continued data collection is vital. The system is under continuous appraisal. Its flexibility allows amendment of existing functions and development of new applications. It has not yet completely replaced manual charting but has reduced the amount of clerical work required of the medical and nursing staff. Although success of such a project is difficult to gauge objectively, the fact that this system has been operational in our RICU for five years and is now an accepted part of unit routine, suggests that the initial aims have been achieved.

References

Davis PD, Kenny GNC, Campbell D (1982) On-line analysis of respiratory function with a microcomputer. In: Paul JP, Jordan MM, Ferguson-Pell MW, Andrews BJ (eds.). Computing in medicine. Macmillan, London, pp. 52–56

Glaeser DH, Thomas LJ (1975) Computer monitoring in patient care. Ann Rev Biophys Bioeng 4: 449–476

Jenkins MA, Cheezum L, Essick V (1968) Clinical patient management and the integrated health care system. Med Instrum 12: 217–221

Kenny GNC, Campbell D (1982) Microcomputer assisted cardiovascular monitoring. In: Paul JP, Jordan MM, Ferguson-Pell MW, Andrews BJ (eds.). Computing in medicine. Macmillan, London, pp. 27–30

Kenny GNC, Davis PD (1983) Computer techniques in critical care medicine. In: Ledingham IMcA, Hanning, CD (eds.) Recent advances in critical care medicine. Churchill-Livingstone, Edinburgh, pp. 197–209

Miller J, Preston TD, Dann PE, Bailey JS, Tobin G (1978) Charting versus computing. Nurs Times 74: 1423–1425

Osborne JJ, Beaumont JO, Raison J, Jerome R, Gerbode F (1968) Measuring and monitoring of the acutely ill patient by digital computer. Surgery 64: 1057–1070

Phillips GD, Gordon AJ, Cousins MJ (1982) Computer based monitoring and data analysis in anaesthesia and intensive care. Anaesthes Intensive Care 10: 223

Reid JA, Kenny GNC (1987) Evaluation of closed-loop control of arterial blood pressure after cardiopulmonary bypass. Br J Anaesth 57: 247–255

Sheppard LC (1979) The computer in the care of the critically ill patient. Proc Inst Electron Electric Eng 67: 1300–1306

Stewart JSS (1982) Patient monitoring by computer:– large or small? In: Paul JP, Jordan MM, Ferguson-Pell MW, Andrews BJ (eds.) Computing in medicine. Macmillan, London, pp. 27–30

7 Clinical Data Capture using a Pressure Sensitive Graphics Pad – APACHE Scoring in the Intensive Therapy Unit

R.G. Jones, P.O. Collinson, M. Howes and G. Boran

Introduction

The success or failure of any computer application rests heavily on user acceptance. The increasing power and decreasing cost and size of computer facilities have led to the widespread promotion of microcomputers in the medical field for a variety of applications. However, full realisation of the computer's potential has yet to be made due, in part, to deficiencies in the human–computer interface (Schneiderman 1986). The standard software interface uses a QWERTY keyboard, usually combined with a series of menus. Unfortunately, this often proves unacceptable in clinical situations. Medical users (doctors and nurses) are rarely familiar with keyboards and few are skilled typists. Ergonomic constraints limit the suitability of keyboard data entry in clinical situations. Keyboards are not portable, requiring that the application be tied to a particular location, or that bulky equipment (such as a lap-portable computer) is brought into the crowded clinical environment. Shortliffe (1987), principal developer of ONCOCIN, Stanford University's expert system for cancer therapy management, has remarked that users' difficulties with keyboards has been one of the major hindrances for the acceptance of computer solutions for clinical problems. Mouse-driven software, light-pens and touch screens have been advocated as alternatives but these rely on the combination of a screen and QWERTY keyboard and suffer from the same lack of portability. Small hand-held terminals are available, such as the PSION Organiser (Psion, London, UK), and can be used for remote data capture. But they still have an alphanumeric keyboard and in our experience suffer from drawbacks similar to those of the QWERTY keyboard.

Recognising the need for rapid and cost-effective data entry we have developed a novel approach using a pressure-sensitive pad as the interface hardware, married to keyboards based on paper proformas. This approach closely simulates normal clinical practice, with bedside data capture, as the device is portable.

Also, because a paper record is made simultaneously with the electronic entry, it complements current methods of record keeping. As an example of its use we describe an application which involves the capture and analysis of data at the bedside in the intensive therapy unit (ITU).

The Clinical Application

The APACHE II (*A*cute *P*hysiological *A*ssessment with *C*hronic *H*ealth *E*valuation, Knaus et al. 1985) scoring system has been developed in the USA as a clinical audit tool (Morgan and Branthwaite 1986; Editorial 1986). Weighted scores are derived from a set of physiological, demographic and neurological measurements made on patients, the sum of these scores constituting the APACHE II score. Table 7.1 lists the parameters used and Table 7.2 indicates how the weighted scores are derived, using temperature as an example. The magnitude of the total score for an individual patient correlates with the severity of illness and high scores are a predictor of likely fatal outcome.

Table 7.1. Parameters used to calculate the APACHE II score in an individual patient

Age
Chronic health score (based on mode of admission to ITU;
    presence of organ failure or immunosuppression)
Body temperature
Heart rate
Respiratory rate
Arterial oxygenation
Arterial pH
Plasma sodium
Plasma potassium
Plasma creatinine
Haematocrit
White cell count
Glasgow coma score

Table 7.2. The data intervals for temperature and the derived weighted scores assigned under the APACHE II system. Note that the scores rise as the temperature deviates from the normal range

Temperature (°C)	Score (points)
>41	4
39.0–40.9	3
38.5–38.9	1
36.0–38.4	0
34.0–35.9	1
32.0–33.9	2
30.0–31.9	3
<29.9	4

The introduction of this scoring system to the ITU highlights the problems which accompany the expansion of information technology into clinical medicine. The logging of the data is seen as an increase in workload by ITU staff since collection and calculation of the scores by hand is laborious and time-consuming. This detracts from traditional patient care. Manual calculation is prone to error, and provides an ideal model against which to test the application of novel techniques of computerised data capture. The computational task is relatively trivial: to log the necessary parameters and to convert these into weighted scores and derive the total. The problem for the information technologist is to achieve this in a manner which is efficient, has high user acceptability and is ergonomically satisfactory.

System Description

The system has at its core a relational database written in PASCAL (Turbo Pascal, Borland International, Scotts Valley, California, USA) running on an IBM-PC compatible microcomputer. Its purpose is to store patient demographic details and the APACHE II scores. Although the primary aim of our work has been to evaluate the effectiveness of alternative keyboard devices in the clinical environment, we considered that this would only be possible in the context of a fully functional computer system. Hence, the database provides a number of valuable ward functions. These include bed-state reporting facilities compatible with the requirements of the current Korner minimum dataset (DHSS 1983) since the ability to automate routine work offers the nursing staff an immediate incentive to use the system. The program also produces patient labels, ward discharge and patient summaries as well as allowing users to search selectively for subgroups of patients. In addition, facilities are included for links to external packages, such as the statistical package OXSTAT (Medstat Ltd, Nottingham, UK), to allow for more sophisticated data analysis.

The host microcomputer software itself has been written with the untrained user in mind. The interface has been kept as simple as possible with a consistent approach to the positioning of screen messages and judicious use of colour to distinguish data from prompts, labels and instructions. Context-sensitive help is also provided through the use of pop-up prompt screens and menus, again colour coded. In this way the need for the user to consult manuals or aides memoire is minimised.

Using this basic system we have been able to test different methods of entering the APACHE data set. Because the data remain constant, and the objective is to derive the final APACHE score, direct comparisons of speed, error rates and subjective appreciation of the different methods have been possible. Thus, the graphics pad method has been compared with QWERTY keyboard input and a simple mouse-driven pull-down menu interface.

Graphics Pad Hardware

The graphics pad (Perex Multipad, Perex Engineering, Reading) consists of a pressure-sensitive surface with a working area of 211 × 297 mm (A4 paper size)

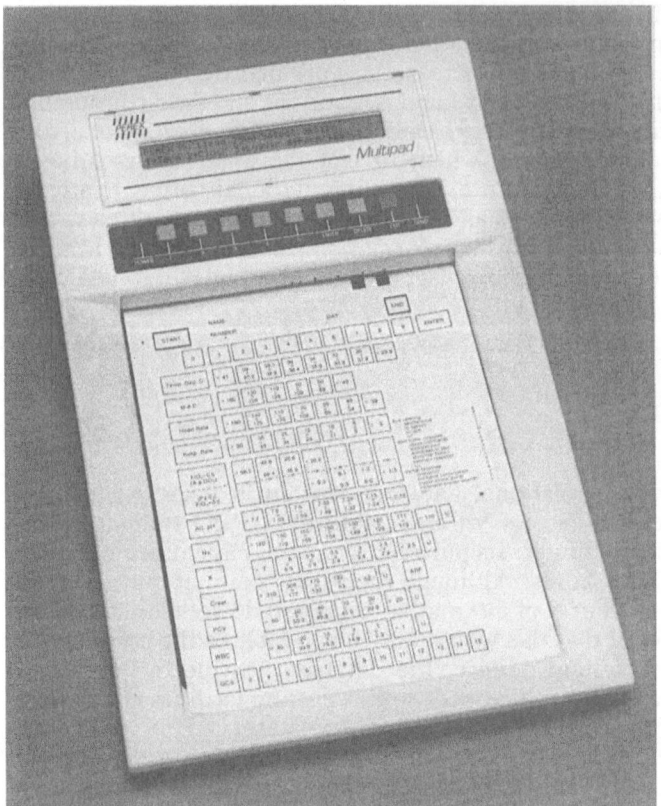

Fig. 7.1. The Perex Multipad. Note the A4-size digitising surface, the LCD screen and the panel of control buttons.

(Fig. 7.1). The pad responds to point pressure, such as that made by a pen. An in-built programmable 48 K RAM microprocesser identifies the coordinates of the point and converts them into meaningful data items. These can be stored and later transmitted to a host microcomputer via an RS232 serial interface. The entire unit measures 430 × 285 × 35 mm and weighs 2.6 kg. Its built-in rechargeable power supply enables several hours of portable use. For communication with users the unit has a two-line, 40-character liquid crystal display panel.

Before the pad can be used in an application a suitable keyboard must be designed and the pad programmed to recognise it and respond appropriately. Keyboards are designed on A4 paper, usually using a word processor, and consist of a number of boxes which act as the "keys". The unit is programmed to recognise the keyboard through an 8-bit bar code at the top right of the sheet allowing up to 255 different keyboards to be specified and used interchangeably on the same pad. By the use of software built into the pad the position of each of the boxes is defined. Once this is done, it is possible to link data items to the boxes. In its simplest form, activating a key can result in a single character or digit being stored in the pad memory. In practice, longer complex strings or codes are usually used, allowing a single key press to enter a large amount of data.

Importantly, a variety of functions may be associated with the keys so that sophisticated data-capture procedures can be set up. These functions include prompts to the user for further action, date and time stamping of data entries, control of the sequence of allowable key entries and simple arithmetic tallying to count the frequencies of certain key entries. In this way data errors may be minimised and data verification becomes virtually automatic. A more detailed description of the programming procedure is given in another chapter of this book (Chap. 9).

Data Entry – a Practical Example

Knaus et al. (1985) originally represented the data set of their APACHE II scoring system as a 9×12 matrix, each row corresponding to a parameter and each column to the data intervals. Apache point scores could then be assigned according to the intervals in which the individual data items lay. Such an approach is ideally suited to data entry using the graphics pad and we simply converted Knaus's matrix into a keyboard overlay (Figs. 7.2, 7.3).

After inserting the paper keyboard, data entry is begun by pressing the START key and the user is prompted to enter the patient's identification number. The date is recorded automatically by the pad from its real-time clock but it can be entered by the user if needed. Thereafter data are entered by ticking the boxes corresponding to the physiological measurements, the response being held in memory in the pad. For example, on ticking the pH box "7.33–7.49" the pad displays and stores "Data 7.33–7.49 APS 0". Data entry is terminated by pressing the END key. Scores can subsequently be checked and edited in the pad memory. Because data for each patient are uniquely identified by the hospital number, the scores for several patients can be collected during one ward round and later transferred to the microcomputer. Here they are automatically incorporated into the appropriate records of the database.

Advantages and Disadvantages

In practice we have identified several major advantages of the pad. First, data entry is by a familiar method, pen on paper. This has resulted in high acceptability, especially among staff potentially hostile to computer use. It is a common complaint that medical and nursing staff did not train "to become typists". Continuing to use existing skills has clear advantages, reflected in this case by the shorter training periods required for pad usage compared to QWERTY keyboard data entry. Error-free data entry was achieved after only two trials by pad users, in contrast to eight trials for users of the conventional keyboard. Second, it was notable that fewer errors were made using the pad compared to the keyboard, particularly errors related to the procedural aspects of data entry, e.g. pressing keys in incorrect sequence or making entries out of order. A verifiable paper copy of the entered data is generated immediately and can be stored. This is clearly an important consideration as it covers some medico-legal requirements. Thirdly, speed of data entry may be increased. Using the pad,

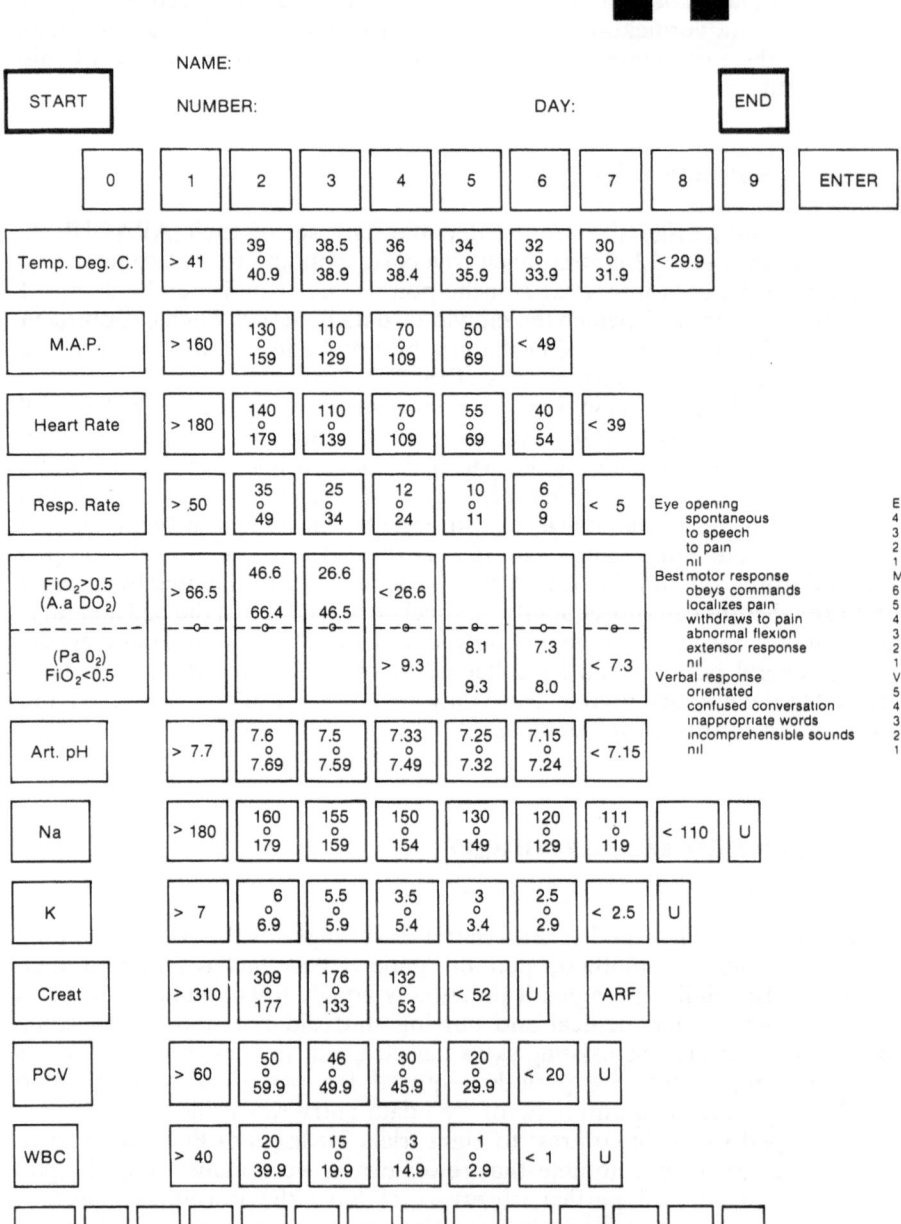

Fig. 7.2. The A4-size keyboard used for the capture of APACHE II scores. Note the bar code at the top right of the sheet.

Temp. Deg. C.	> 41	39 o 40.9	38.5 o 38.9	36 o 38.4	34 o 35.9	32 o 33.9	30 o 31.9	< 29.9

Fig. 7.3. Close-up of pad overlay for APACHE II scoring, showing keys used for entry of temperature scores. Note the small central targets.

it is possible to input a complete Apache II data set in 1 minute if the data are all available. We have found that it may take inexperienced users up to 20 minutes per patient to generate an Apache II score by typing data into the patient database. Practised users show little difference in speed between the keyboard and the pad. Finally, the pad is portable. This is probably its single most important attribute as data acquisition is possible at the patient's bedside where most of the charts are kept.

Similar comparisons have been possible for mouse-driven capture of Apache II data. The mouse interface fares badly in comparison to both the pad and the keyboard. Although accurate, it proves unacceptably slow and cumbersome and new users take a long time to become familiar with its use. Like the keyboard, no immediate hard copy record is produced and, again, it is not portable.

However, like all computer devices, the pad has its limitations. The system discussed above uses a tick box method of data entry which is most suitable for grouped data such as Apache scores. Though, it can also be used to capture interval data, we have found it performs less well when discrete numbers or free text must be entered. We are currently exploring other possibilities such as the use of analogue scales where absolute accuracy is not of critical importance, for example in fluid balance and total parenteral nutrition monitoring. Physically there are also some problems; it is only just portable, since carrying an object which weighs 2.6 kg for long periods can be quite tiring. The bar-code reader for keyboard recognition also tends to be unreliable and, although a minor problem technically, this can be extremely inconvenient. Lastly, although the in-built custom software allows clever input systems to be designed, it is cumbersome to program and lacks the flexibility of a standard high-level language such as PASCAL. Ideally, we would like to see the device re-engineered to the size and weight of an ordinary clipboard and to have included in it a microcomputer running a standard operating system such as MS–DOS (Microsoft Inc, Reading, UK). Sophisticated software could then be developed on standard personal computers and downloaded into the device for use. As hand-writing encoders are now becoming a reality the inclusion of this capability would produce a keyboard with a multitude of applications limited only be the imagination of its users. Indeed, such a device could well be made now using existing components.

Conclusions

Our work with the graphics pad has demonstrated that alternative data capture techniques can make computer systems more acceptable to clinical users. It is important to remember that clever functions performed by using a microcomputer will only be of benefit if users find them accessible and complementary to their normal working practice. A critical component in this respect is the human–computer interface, the design of which should take account of the essential human factors of the interaction (Foley et al. 1984). It is unlikely that any one method of interaction will provide a universal solution to all design problems but the pad described above meets many of the putative requirements of the clinical computer interface.

References

D.H.S.S. (1983) First report of the steering group on health services information. (Chairman, E Korner). HMSO, London.

Editorial (1986) TPN and APACHE. Lancet i: 1478

Foley J, Wallace V, Chan P (1984) The human factors of computer graphics interaction techniques. IEEE Computer Graphics and Applications, 4: 13–48

Knaus WA, Draper EA, Wagner DP, Zimmerman JE (1985) APACHE II: a severity of disease classification system. Crit Care Med 13: 818–829

Morgan CJ, Branthwaite MA (1986) Severity scoring in intensive care. Br Med J 292: 1546

Schneiderman B (1986) Designing the user interface. Addison-Wesley, Reading, Mass

Shortliffe, EH (1987) Computer programs to support clinical decision making. JAMA 258: 61–66

8 Implementation and Clinical Applications of a Computerised Fluid and Electrolyte Balance and Nutritional Management System

G. Boran, P. Collinson, R. Jones and D. Cramp

Introduction

Calculations of fluid balance have played an important role in the monitoring of fluid therapy and volume status for many years, and they constitute an essential part of the management of critically ill patients. The simplest form of calculation subtracts the total measured fluid losses from the total fluid volumes administered, resulting in a balance figure which implies fluid overload when positive (i.e. input exceeds output) and fluid deficit when negative.

Although these calculations are mathematically simple, they demand considerable time and attention from those responsible for maintaining fluid balance charts. Furthermore, the results of such calculations are limited to the management of fluid volume status. Additional calculations can be made to reflect water, sodium, potassium and nitrogen balance and energy intake, provided the composition of all administered fluid, drugs and feeding regimens is known, and appropriate measurements are made on the daily losses. Derivation of these data extends the applications of fluid balance calculations to the management of electrolyte disorders. Energy intake and nitrogen balance may be used to monitor nutritional therapy, classically in total parenteral nutrition but also during enteral feeding.

Like most indices of fluid and electrolyte balance, fluid balance data are most useful when performed on a regular basis – usually daily for critically ill patients. Daily calculations allow trend detection and derivation of cumulative figures representing, for instance, cumulative potassium balance. Such detailed calculations are not feasible by manual methods but are ideally suited to automated methods, particularly as powerful inexpensive microcomputers are now so readily available.

Microcomputers have resulted in a revival of interest in sequential balance studies because they calculate precise daily and cumulative balance data and can present the results by the use of graphical methods to facilitate trend detection. Computerised systems also eliminate mathematical errors, which tend to increase in proportion to the amount and complexity of data in manual systems. Of course, errors in the charting of administered fluids or in the measurement of fluid losses, and uncertainties concerning insensible losses, affect the accuracy of computerised systems as well as manual systems for fluid balance. Appropriate use of computer technology, with attention to effective means of data input, will minimise errors in the recording of data and will liberate the nurse in the intensive therapy unit (ITU) from secretarial tasks to devote more time to patient care.

In the following discussion, the specification and details of implementation will be presented for a fluid balance system currently in use in critical care environments. Clinical applications made possible by continuous daily monitoring will be discussed, together with a consideration of the limitations of balance studies and prospects for further development.

Specification

We have developed a combined fluid balance and nutritional management system for use in ITUs, metabolic wards and other critical care environments. The total parenteral nutrition (TPN) prescription component of the system is described elsewhere (see Chap. 9) and the following discussion refers to the fluid balance component.

Hardware Requirements

Hardware requirements are fulfilled by any standard IBM-compatible microcomputer using the Intel 8086, 8088, 80286 or 80386 microprocessors, or certain others such as the NEC V20. The system runs under the MS–DOS or PC–DOS operating systems. Compatibility will be maintained with the new OS/2 operating system recently announced by the Microsoft Corporation. IBM compatibility was chosen because of the widespread availability of inexpensive machines affording a high level of software portability. At least 384 kilobytes of random access memory should be available and a 20-Mbyte hard disc storage facility is advisable. A colour graphics monitor facilitates optimal presentation of data and a fast dot-matrix printer is required to produce the written reports and histogram plots. The keyboard may be used to enter data, but we have developed an additional method of data entry using a portable low-resolution graphics tablet (Perex Multipad, Perex Engineering Limited, Reading, UK). This device is fully described elsewhere (see Chap. 9).

Software

The source code was written and compiled using the QUICKBASIC compiler version 2 (Microsoft Corporation), a semi-structured version of the traditional

BASIC language. Up to ten active patients are allowed and each patient may be monitored for up to 2 months. This has proven satisfactory for most purposes.

Implementation

Data are entered by keyboard or by using the graphics tablet. The system calculates the balance figures by summating the water, sodium, potassium, nitrogen and energy content of the fluid, drug and nutritional therapies and then subtracting the measured or estimated quantities of water, sodium, potassium and nitrogen in urine and other fluid losses. Results are then displayed on the monitor by both graphical and numerical techniques, and printed copies of the output are generated.

Keyboard Method of Data Entry

In the keyboard method of data entry, the user selects the appropriate input fluids from a menu displaying the names of up to 50 fluid, drug, and nutritional therapies. The volumes may be entered either as a daily total or as a series of hourly totals. Full error-trapping is performed on all input and certain preset physiological limits must be observed. The urine and other losses are entered in a separate menu. Urine urea is required to calculate nitrogen losses. Urine losses can be entered as daily totals. Alternatively, the electrolytes may be entered as concentrations, provided a daily urine volume is supplied. Abnormal losses by other routes are currently entered as single figures representing daily losses of water, sodium and potassium. Insensible water loss and the patient's body weight, temperature and the day-to-day change in plasma urea concentration are also entered via the output menu. Once all data are entered, control passes to the calculation procedures.

Non-Keyboard Method of Data Entry

An additional software interface had to be developed to accommodate data entry using the Perex graphics tablet (Multipad). The Multipad provides a rapid, convenient and reliable method of entering data which are selected from short lists of alternatives and is extensively used in the TPN component of this system (see Chap. 9). Since fluid volumes usually cannot be easily banded into short lists of alternatives, the use of the Multipad in the fluid balance component is limited to selection of input and output fluids. Nevertheless, the fluid balance interface has been developed on a trial basis and it permits some improvements over the keyboard method since the portable Multipad, unlike the host microcomputer, can be brought to the bedside to enter data on several patients in batch mode.

When using the Multipad for fluid balance calculations, a sheet of A4 paper with boxes drawn to represent the various fluids is placed as an overlay on the device's pressure-sensitive pad. Data are stored for eventual transmission to the host computer in response to pressure over the appropriate box. All commonly used fluid or nutritional therapies and categories of measured loss (e.g. urine, nasogastric) are allocated to individual boxes and can be activated by a single light application of pressure from a pen. Boxes must also be allocated to represent the numbers zero to nine as a numerical keypad so that the volumes may be entered on the Multipad, exactly as they are entered using the keyboard. Even with these limitations, the Multipad can accelerate the rate of data entry.

Since the successful implementation of non-keyboard methods of data entry depends as much on causing minimal disruption of existing work practices as on improving the speed and reliability of data entry, more sophisticated interfaces are currently being examined. For instance, the use of written language interfaces may succeed in trapping a patient's fluid data for later computer processing as the ITU nurse writes it on the patient's fluid chart, thus simultaneously generating a computer record and an original hand-written record to conform with existing work practices.

Insensible Water Loss

Insensible water loss varies according to the patient's body temperature, respiratory rate and body surface area. Respiratory rate is maintained fairly constant in ventilated patients and gross fluctuations in surface area probably do not occur. Hence, it seems reasonable to use a constant figure for basal insensible water loss in most patients. This is currently preset to 500 ml/day but can be easily changed by the user if thought necessary.

However, temperature fluctuations are likely to produce large changes in insensible water loss. While it is impossible to determine insensible losses precisely, algorithms have been empirically derived relating changes in body temperature in pyrexial patients to increases in water loss over the basal insensible losses. One such algorithm (Eqn. 8.1) has been implemented in this system.

$$\text{Correction} = W \times t \times 7.142 \qquad\qquad \text{Eqn. 8.1}$$

The patient's body weight (W (kg)) and temperature increase over 37.5 °C (t (°C)) must be supplied to make this correction, which is added to the basal insensible loss. The correction amounts to approximately 500 ml per degree rise in temperature for a 70 kg patient and has been found to be satisfactory in practice.

Nitrogen Balance Correction Factor

Increases in plasma-urea concentration result in an underestimation of protein catabolism because urinary nitrogen losses are falsely low. An empirically derived algorithm (Eqn. 8.2) which calculates a nitrogen balance correction factor (NBF (g/day)), has therefore been introduced.

$$\text{NBF} = P \times W \times 0.0168 \qquad\qquad \text{Eqn. 8.2}$$

The correction factor is positive if plasma-urea concentration has increased and the result is subtracted from overall nitrogen balance. Use of this algorithm is entirely optional. It requires as input the change in plasma-urea concentration (P (mmol/l)) and the body weight (W (kg)). The correction amounts to approximately 1 g nitrogen per mmol increase in plasma urea concentration for a 70 kg patient.

Calculation of Balance Data

During the calculation procedure, the system references a file from which it determines the water, sodium, potassium, nitrogen and energy composition of up to 50 possible fluid, drug and nutritional therapies which may have been entered. The daily urinary urea losses are converted to grams of nitrogen in order to determine the nitrogen losses. The appropriate insensible water loss is calculated and so is the nitrogen balance correction factor. These are treated in the calculation as extra sources of water and nitrogen loss, respectively. Subtraction of total outputs from total inputs for each of water, sodium, potassium and nitrogen yields the balance figures. At present, no attempt is made to determine energy balance: only energy intake is reported. Water balance is reported in ml/ day, potassium and sodium in mmol/day, nitrogen in g/day and energy intake in kJ/day. Cumulative water, sodium, potassium and nitrogen balances as functions of time are calculated by adding the individual data for each available day.

Compatibility with the TPN Prescription Component

Fluids and nutritional therapies prescribed for a patient using the TPN prescription component are automatically entered as input fluids for the purposes of the fluid balance component. Balance data are generated as soon as the daily losses are entered either through the Multipad or via the keyboard. Modifications are allowed in case the fluid volumes administered differ from those prescribed.

Presentation of Results

Newly entered data may be repeatedly scrutinised and corrected on the monitor before the balance figures are finally calculated and displayed. All correction factors in use are clearly shown. Previously filed data may also be examined in this way and recalculated and updated if necessary. Histograms of each type of balance information can be plotted as a function of time and displayed on the monitor or printer. These are particularly useful for trend detection and are easier to assimilate than are numerical data. Printed output is more useful, however, since the data may then be displayed by the bedside with the patient's fluid charts where they are likely to be considered in patient management. Copies are also required for the medical records. Accordingly, great emphasis is put on a readable print-out in our system. Each patient receives a report consisting of graphical and numerical representations of the balance data as a function of time. The contribution of intake and losses to the daily and cumulative balance figures are also shown. Hence, sodium and potassium balances are split into intake (mmol/day) and output (mmol/day). Water intake and output are reported as ml/ day and nitrogen intake as g/day.

Clinical Applications

The following sections outline our experience of the use of fluid, electrolyte and nutritional balance data over a 2-year development period.

Balance Data in Hypernatraemia

Water balance can be used to monitor fluid therapy in much the same way as fluid balance, but the two are not numerically equal. The discrepancy between water and fluid balance is particularly obvious in patients receiving blood or "Intralipid" solutions where the aqueous content is significantly less than the administered volume. For instance, "Intralipid 20%" is 75% and whole blood 55% aqueous by volume.

Patients with hypernatraemia due to water deficiency show negative water balance. Whether this is a result of poor intake or excessive losses will be obvious from the intake/output figures if not from more direct clinical examination. Since urinary sodium losses are minimal in such patients, sodium balance may be positive, depending on sodium intake and the extent of other losses. Sodium output is usually negligible unless the abnormal routes are active.

In hypernatraemia due to sodium excess, clearly positive sodium balance without negative water balance is usually found. Its distinction from water deficiency may be more obvious after examining the trends of the previous few days. Sodium intake and output data may reveal excessive intake, decreased output, or a mixture of both. Some patients show a combination of clearly positive sodium balance with negative water balance, implying that a combination of water deficiency and sodium excess is present. Cumulative water and sodium balance may reflect changes in total body water and sodium in these patients. In any event, great care is advisable in their interpretation because of the uncertainties surrounding insensible water losses.

The effects of therapy for hypernatraemia can be monitored. Administration of water gradually restores daily water balance data to equilibrium (i.e. nearly to 0 ml/day) as plasma sodium concentrations normalise. Likewise, sodium restriction in sodium excess states can be monitored. The cumulative figures also reflect therapeutic manoeuvres. Balance data appear to be predictors of frank hypernatraemia in some patients. Negative water balances have been seen together with normal but climbing plasma sodium concentrations for a few days before hypernatraemia develops.

Balance Data in Hyponatraemia

Hyponatraemia is usually due to water excess and less often to sodium deficiency. In patients who are hyponatraemic because of the administration of a net hypotonic fluid regime, positive water balance is seen. The therapeutic effect of fluid restriction or isotonic fluid administration can be monitored using balance data as well as the plasma sodium concentration.

Hyponatraemic patients with large renal or extra-renal sodium losses or who are receiving diuretics may show negative sodium balances with large sodium output figures. Water balance in these patients depends on water intake and losses, but low water output data are not uncommon particularly if hypovolaemia supervenes.

Balance Data in Potassium Disorders

Plasma potassium concentration is a poor indicator of total body potassium and can be maintained in the reference range even when total body potassium

Table 8.1. Potassium balance (BAL), intake (IN) and output (OUT) data in mmol/day. Histogram shows balance data in mmol/day. [K]: plasma potassium concentrations in mmol/l (added manually)

Date	−300	0	+300	Potassium balance data			
				BAL	IN	OUT	[K]
17/07/87	***I			−62	21	83	4.4
18/07/87	***I			−56	19	75	3.1
19/07/87	I*			17	154	137	2.8
20/07/87	I**			31	160	129	2.7
21/07/87	I**			47	171	124	3.1
22/07/87	******I			−120	83	203	3.1
23/07/87	******I			−114	64	178	3.6
24/07/87	*******I			−133	0	133	4.2
25/07/87	*******I			−142	0	142	3.2
26/07/87	********I			−154	0	154	2.8
27/07/87	****I			−77	0	77	3.4
28/07/87	**I			−49	22	71	3.7
29/07/87	***I			−63	23	86	4.3
30/07/87	**I			−45	26	71	4.0
31/07/87	**I			−34	26	60	4.1
01/08/87	*I			−17	43	60	4.2
02/08/87	**I			−40	51	91	4.4
03/08/87	**I			−43	51	94	3.8
04/08/87	*****I			−96	39	135	3.7
05/08/87	*******I			−137	0	137	7.4
06/08/87	*****I			−107	0	107	2.6
07/08/87		I**		35	176	141	3.0
08/08/87		I*****		105	209	104	3.3
09/08/87		I******		126	264	138	3.9
10/08/87	**I			−45	232	277	3.7
11/08/87	*I			−20	116	136	5.1
Cumulative balance (mmol)				−1193	1950	3143	

deficiency is present. This is particularly the case in acidotic or hypovolaemic patients. We have observed that many patients who have negative potassium balance but are normokalaemic will manifest intermittent or frank hypokalaemia at a later stage, unless potassium supplements are given to correct the deficit. Cumulative potassium balance may reflect changes in total body potassium, provided the patient's muscle mass is stable over the period of observation. Potassium supplementation can be monitored using the daily and cumulative figures.

In patients with secondary hyperaldosteronism, persistent negative potassium balance may be accompanied by positive sodium balance and the hypernatraemia of sodium excess. This disorder is not uncommon in postoperative ITU patients, particularly those with hepatic dysfunction.

Potassium balance data generated by our system for such a patient are shown in Table 8.1, with the plasma potassium concentrations added for comparison. Consistently negative daily and cumulative potassium balance with relatively large potassium output is evident from the date of admission (17/07/87). Marked hypokalaemia developed on at least two occasions (26/07/87 and 6/08/87) following reductions in potassium intake. Plasma potassium concentrations were generally normal in spite of a cumulative negative potassium balance of 1193 mmol, which corresponds to a loss of about one-third of total body potassium.

Table 8.2. Sodium balance (BAL), intake (IN) and output (OUT) data in mmol/day. Histogram shows balance data in mmol/day. [Na]: plasma sodium concentrations in mmol/l (added manually)

Date	−300	0	+300	Sodium balance data			
				BAL	IN	OUT	[Na]
17/07/87		I******************		352	660	308	143
18/07/87		I***********		225	532	307	144
19/07/87		I*******		146	347	201	142
20/07/87		***I		−58	85	143	146
21/07/87		I*		21	228	207	155
22/07/87		*********I		−179	160	339	156
23/07/87		I**		36	145	109	159
24/07/87		************I		−211	3	214	162
25/07/87		*******I		−139	112	251	160
26/07/87		****I		−89	104	193	158
27/07/87		I*		19	53	34	159
28/07/87		I**		42	44	2	150
29/07/87		I*****		95	97	2	151
30/07/87		I***		51	53	2	145
31/07/87		I**		46	53	7	143
01/08/87		I****		78	85	7	139
02/08/87		I*****		101	102	1	139
03/08/87		I*****		98	103	5	144
04/08/87		I		−4	0	4	149
05/08/87		I		−6	0	6	151
06/08/87		I		−4	0	4	145
07/08/87		I		−4	0	4	145
08/08/87		I*		25	28	3	143
09/08/87		I		−4	0	4	152
10/08/87		I		3	12	9	149
11/08/87		I**		40	44	4	147
Cumulative balance (mmol)				680	3050	2370	

Table 8.2 shows sodium balance (with plasma sodium concentrations added) and Table 8.3 water balance data for this patient. Low sodium output accompanied by positive sodium balance and episodes of hypernatraemia (Table 8.2) are present from 27/07/87. Although water balance (Table 8.3) is generally positive after 27/07/87, an episode of negative water balance (1/08/87 to 3/08/87) contributed to the hypernatraemia.

Balance Data in Oedematous States

Patients with interstitial fluid accumulation frequently show positive daily and cumulative water balance. Cautious interpretation of the cumulative figure may indicate the volume of retained fluid, and is usually greater than 5 l when oedema is palpable clinically. However, any errors in the daily insensible water losses (particularly those consistently biased in one direction) are additive and lead to problems of interpretation.

Table 8.3. Water balance (BAL), intake (IN) and output (OUT) data in ml/day. Histogram shows balance data in ml/day.

Date	−2500	0	+2500	Water balance data		
				BAL	IN	OUT
17/07/87		I********		1306	5173	3867
18/07/87		I**********		1675	5298	3623
19/07/87		I		80	4060	3980
20/07/87		*I		−244	3586	3830
21/07/87		**I		−288	3904	4192
22/07/87	****************I			−2612	3659	6271
23/07/87		****I		−707	2900	3607
24/07/87		*******I		−1247	2983	4230
25/07/87		*I		−87	3698	3785
26/07/87		I**		319	3901	3582
27/07/87		I********		1354	3752	2398
28/07/87		I*****		825	3335	2510
29/07/87		I************		1996	3701	1705
30/07/87		I***		629	3589	2960
31/07/87		I****************		2651	4703	2052
01/08/87		***I		−465	3329	3794
02/08/87		**I		−257	2698	2955
03/08/87		*******I		−1137	2639	3776
04/08/87		I*****************		2815	5972	3157
05/08/87		I**		308	3748	3440
06/08/87		I***		539	3924	3385
07/08/87		****I		−631	2744	3375
08/08/87		I*		159	3642	3483
09/08/87		*I		−102	3826	3928
10/08/87		I*		86	3503	3417
11/08/87		I********		1417	4081	2664
Cumulative balance (ml)				8382	98348	89966

Balance Data in Nutritional Monitoring

Nitrogen balance and energy intake may be used to monitor parenteral and enteral nutrition and may affect subsequent TPN prescriptions made by using the TPN prescription component of this system.

Conclusion

We have found this system to be a valuable tool in the management of fluid balance and nutritional problems in critically ill patients. New approaches to the man–machine interface are under assessment, as are knowledge-based systems to analyse and interpret the data. Our intention is to produce friendly unobtrusive systems which will support the clinician and nurse, and ultimately result in improved patient care.

9 A Computer-Based System for Total Parenteral Prescription at the Bedside

P.O. Collinson, G.R. Boran and R.G. Jones

Introduction

Total parenteral nutrition (TPN) is an integral part of the management of patients with gastrointestinal failure. This is a complex and high-cost area of medicine requiring good record keeping. For the clinician the nutritional regime must be integrated with the overall fluid, nitrogen and energy balance strategy for the patient. This requires calculation of the composition of the feeding regimen and its incorporation into balance calculations. This is especially true for those patients in critical care beds where strict monitoring of fluid balance is essential. Calculation and presentation of water, electrolyte, energy and nitrogen balance information is extremely time-consuming when performed manually but ideally suited to a microcomputer-based system. For the TPN nurse the system should keep records of the menus prescribed, the type of intravenous line and nursing procedures performed. For the pharmacist, regimens administered must be monitored for compatibility of components particularly when addition of further electrolytes is performed. Finally, data must be available to the parenteral nutrition team for audit.

System Requirements

We have approached the problem of the prescription of the nutritional regimen and its integration with fluid balance calculation, pharmacy formulation and the patient database. In total parenteral nutrition prescription a menu must be decided and prescribed on the ward. It is then written out in the pharmacy, checked for compatibility of components and formulated. A label for the bag detailing its composition must then be prepared, checked with the menu and affixed to the bag. The bag is then taken to the ward and checked against the prescription on the ward fluid chart before it is administered.

The present system has a number of problems. The same information is written or typed out in different places. This is time-consuming for the prescriber and pharmacist and can result in transcription errors. There is no ward record of the actual composition of the feed: hence the inexperienced clinician may be unaware that it contains an appropriate electrolyte content. This can lead to administration of extra electrolytes such as potassium with possible fatal consequences. Finally, all information is held in different locations on pieces of paper, an unsuitable means for retrospective data analysis.

The requirements are for a system which will allow prescription of a regimen at the bedside with simultaneous electronic capture of the data. It must generate hard copy at this point to allow verification of the data entered at the actual time of prescription. This paper record can then be checked and signed by the prescriber as the prescription itself. The prescription has to be stored for subsequent transfer to the microcomputer. The data communication must be verified, then the data displayed to the user to check prescription content and allow any amendment. The computer should then calculate composition data for the feed and produce the relevant documentation. This should include a prescription menu, a pharmacy worksheet and sticky labels for the bag and ward chart, with positive identification of the patient and the feed for that patient. The system should export this information to the relational database. Finally for the prescriber the system must be less trouble to use than the existing procedures.

The problem with any computer-based system is the entry of data. It is our experience that medical and nursing personnel will use an inconvenient system which has obvious benefit or a convenient system which performs the same role as the preexisting manual system. If neither criterion is fulfilled the system will not be used. To achieve acceptability any proposed system must, as far as possible, mimic normal working practice. In addition we have imposed the requirement for portability and instant hard copy.

We have previously developed a program for fluid balance calculation incorporating TPN data which performs these calculations and contains the necessary data files. Generation of the appropriate documentation and file handling for data export from this software is a relatively simple programming task. The problem is portable data input with verification.

The production of hard copy which can be checked at the stage of data input is difficult by conventional techniques. Portable computers incorporating printers appear to offer a partial solution to this problem. However, they only produce hard copy after data input has occurred and they require a degree of keyboard skill. We have used a portable low resolution graphics tablet, the PEREX Multipad (PEREX Engineering, Reading, Berks) which utilises box ticking with an ordinary pen on paper as the means of data entry. In TPN there is a limited range of formulations for the final prescriptions which are prescribed in unit volumes. Data input is thus of a limited, highly structured dataset. Such a dataset is suitable for this type of data entry.

Hardware and Software

The PEREX multipad is a portable graphics tablet which uses a 211 mm × 297 mm (A4) pressure-sensitive surface as the means of data input. This A4 surface responds to point pressure, such as a pen, but does not respond to large areas of pressure such as a finger or coffee mug. This point pressure is interpreted as an x, y coordinate. This x, y coordinate can be sent directly to a microcomputer host or interpreted by an in-built microcomputer with 48 kbytes of RAM. The unit is able to display up to 80 alphanumeric characters to the user via a two-line 40-character display.

Data input is by box ticking. An overlay with a series of boxes, which act as keys when pressed or ticked, is first laid out on an A4 sheet of paper. The boxes act as keys for program function and for data entry. Pressing an area within the box generates an x, y coordinate which is converted by the software into an instruction, user prompt or meaningful data item. Blank areas of the sheet not coded as boxes are inactive. The overlay is bar coded. This bar code is recognised by a bar-code reader in the unit which can recognise up to 255 different forms. Data entered are stored in memory and can be downloaded to the microcomputer via an RS232C serial interface.

The device is programmed using the pressure-sensitive surface. Box size is first designated by indicating the bottom left then top right corners of the box. The program function for this box is then entered. After the box size has been defined the unit automatically loads an ASCII keyboard onto the pressure-sensitive surface. This is used with a QWERTY keyboard overlay to assign the function for the box (Fig. 9.1), an information or program function. Information boxes act to inform the user by displaying messages as a line of text on the display screen when pressed. This facility may be used to display an instruction to press a function key, the start box, when the unit is switched on. Program functions include, among others, enter, end of record, start, end, automatic date and time stamping of a record, entry of numeric values either as numeric strings or unit quantities and entry of alphanumeric text strings. The data entry can be structured by using two types of command codes. One type guides sequential data entry by allowing prompts to be displayed to the user both during data entry and when the entry is complete. The second type results in all but a series of designated keys being made inactive and requires a set series of operations to be performed before any further data entry may be performed. The program is held as an ASCII file which can be stored on disc for back-up or programming other Multipads.

For TPN prescription an overlay form for the pad was designed on an A4 sheet of paper by using a word processor (Fig. 9.2). All possible components, including electrolyte additions, of the 3-l system are represented, together with the unit volumes used for prescription as a series of boxes. The layout of the sheet follows the order in which the components are usually prescribed. The form includes a linear numeric keypad to allow entry of discrete numeric values. In addition there are three function keys.

The user first writes the patient's name and hospital number on the top of the form for identification and then switches on the unit. The logger mode of the pad is selected and data entry started. The user is prompted to press the Start box. This initiates the data entry. The hospital number is entered to identify the patient record. All data entered at this time for a patient are thus identified as a date and time-stamped record headed by this number. This is the only piece of information requiring the equivalent of key strokes and uses the linear keypad described above. Thereafter data entry is by ticking the relevant box. Hence to prescribe 1000-ml Vamin 14 with electrolytes the Vamin 14 and 1000 ml boxes in that section of the form are ticked. Additives and extra electrolytes are entered as single key operations.

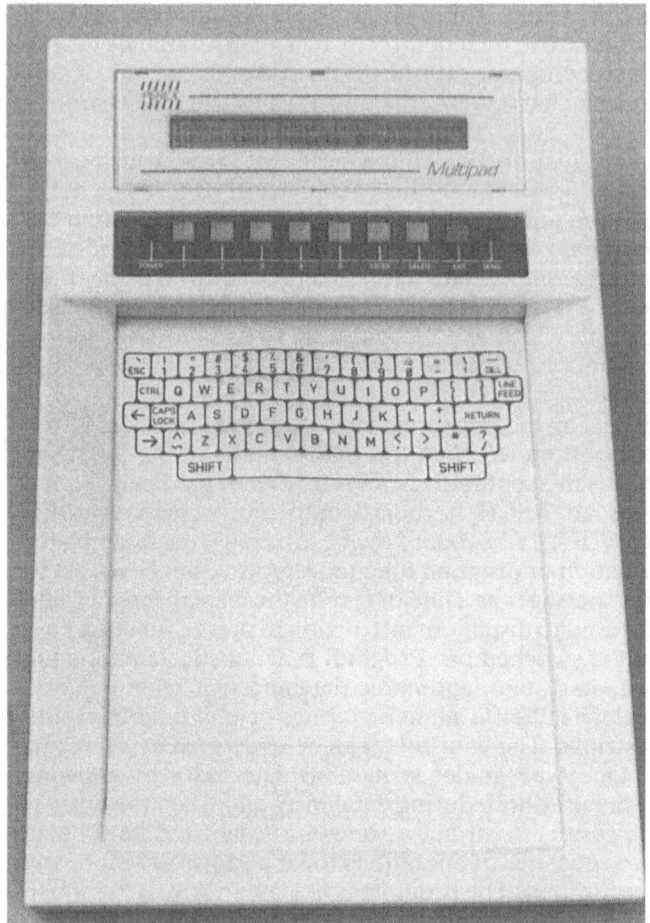

Fig. 9.1. Multipad in programming mode with QWERTY keyboard overlay in position.

As each item is entered it is shown to the prescriber by the display. An incorrect entry or volume can be deleted at the time of entry by using the delete key on the unit. When each item is prescribed the entry is verified by pressing the enter box. The prescription is automatically time and date stamped when data entry is started by software held in the device. The entry is finished by pressing the End box. The paper is then signed and removed as hard copy of the prescription. The data held in memory can be inspected and edited at the bedside should this be required.

The patient record is currently identified by entering the hospital number via the numeric keypad. This can be automated by using a bar-code reader attached to the unit with the hospital number bar coded on the form using a hospital sticky label. Hence, after pressing the start box the bar code would be read and then the boxes ticked, eliminating any need to use a numeric keypad.

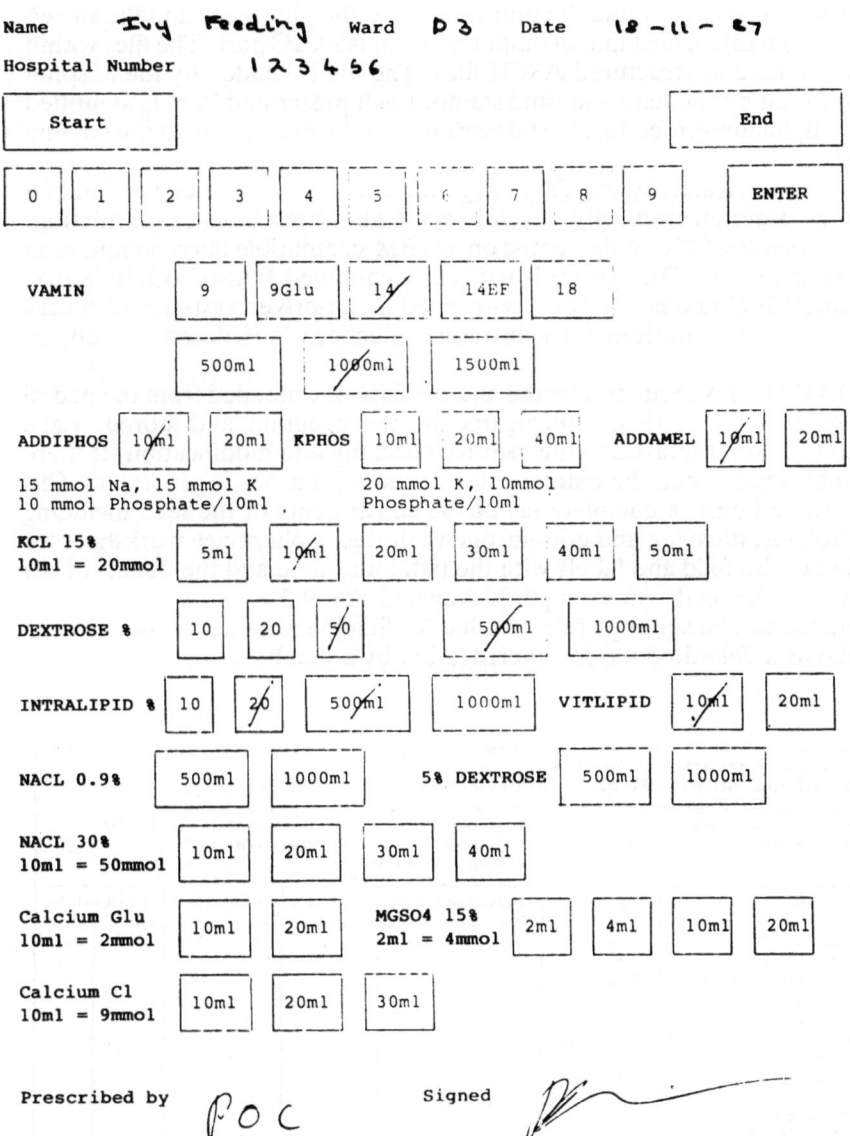

Name Ivy Feeding **Ward** D3 **Date** 18 – 11 – 87
Hospital Number 1 2 3 4 5 6

| Start | | End |

| 0 | 1 | 2 | 3 | 4 | 5 | 6 | 7 | 8 | 9 | ENTER |

VAMIN 9 | 9Glu | 14 | 14EF | 18

500ml | 1000ml | 1500ml

ADDIPHOS 10ml | 20ml **KPHOS** 10ml | 20ml | 40ml **ADDAMEL** 10ml | 20ml

15 mmol Na, 15 mmol K   20 mmol K, 10mmol
10 mmol Phosphate/10ml   Phosphate/10ml

KCL 15%
10ml = 20mmol   5ml | 10ml | 20ml | 30ml | 40ml | 50ml

DEXTROSE %   10 | 20 | 50   500ml | 1000ml

INTRALIPID %   10 | 20 | 500ml | 1000ml   **VITLIPID** 10ml | 20ml

NACL 0.9%   500ml | 1000ml   **5% DEXTROSE** 500ml | 1000ml

NACL 30%
10ml = 50mmol   10ml | 20ml | 30ml | 40ml

Calcium Glu
10ml = 2mmol   10ml | 20ml   **MGSO4 15%**
                              2ml = 4mmol   2ml | 4ml | 10ml | 20ml

Calcium Cl
10ml = 9mmol   10ml | 20ml | 30ml

Prescribed by POC   **Signed**

Fig. 9.2. TPN overlay prescription for a patient.

At the end of the ward round the unit is taken to the pharmacy and the stored data downloaded into a host microcomputer via an RS232C port. The files within the device are held as structured ASCII files. The file is headed by the hospital number followed by the date and time stamp. Each prescribed item is identified by a 3-digit alphanumeric code, a text description of the data and then the volume prescribed.

The file is interrogated by the TPN program. This is an enhanced version of a fluid balance program originally developed for ITU fluid balance calculation. This has been successfully implemented on an IBM-compatible microcomputer in an intensive care unit. The system is written in compiled BASIC (QUICKBA-SIC, Microsoft Inc) and is a fully error-trapped menu-driven system which uses defined single key operations for subroutine selection. It is described fully in Chap. 8.

The LOAD DATA menu is selected and the data downloaded from the pad to a data file. This file is then interrogated by the program and stored. Each prescription is then displayed to the user for checking and modification. If there are no modifications then the data are stored and a print-out is generated. This comprises three items: a complete list of the constituents of the feed including total electrolytes, nitrogen and non-nitrogen calories; a pharmacy worksheet for formulation of the feed and labels with the patient's name and the details of the composition of the feed. An example is shown in Fig. 9.3.

The data file can be subsequently recalled for fluid balance calculation, stored or exported as a delimited file for interrogation by a database.

West Middlesex University Hospital TOTAL PARENTERAL NUTRITION DISPENSING RECORD						
Patient: Ivy Feeding Hosp No: 123456 Batch No:		Ward: Cons: Expiry Date:		TPN Day No: 18/11/87 Prescriber:		
Constituents	Volume	Manufacturer and batch no	Expiry Date	Assembled By	Checked by 1st	2nd
Glucose 50% (ml) Vamin 14 with elec (ml Addiphos (ml) Intralipid 20% (ml) Vitlipid (ml) Addamel (ml) KCl 15% (ml) Solivito (amp) Hydrocortisone (mg) Heparin (U)	500 ml 1000 ml 10 ml 500 ml 10 ml 10 ml 10 ml					
Labels prepared by: checked by:			Bag prepared by: shaken by:			
FINAL CHECK						
Closure and Giving Set	Label and Prescription		Batch Number		Expiry	
PHARMACISTS SIGNATURE:						

Fig. 9.3. Pharmacy worksheet generated following transfer of data to microcomputer for the same patient.

Workplace Evaluation

We have found that this system offers a number of advantages in addition to the data capture facility. The structured nature of the TPN prescription allows more rapid prescription than writing the regime on the fluid chart. We studied 30 prescriptions written by hand or prescribed using the pad. We found the mean time for the hand-written prescription was 125 seconds while for the pad the same prescription averaged 90 seconds. Prescription using the pad also reduced the number of errors. We found that in an average 1-week period with 5 patients fed daily at least two errors would occur. These may be divided into prescription or transcription errors. Prescription errors occurred due to inadvertent omission of one component of the feed, usually an additive. This type of error was confined to the ward prescription chart. It did not occur with the pharmacy or pad prescription since both use a structured form and it is apparent at a glance that an item has been omitted. Transcription errors occurred when the ward and pharmacy prescriptions did not match. This occurred when the pharmacy prescription was written after the round but was not abolished even when the pharmacy and ward charts were written at the same time. No such errors occurred with the pad-based system.

This system uses a familiar mode of data entry, pen on paper; hence the mode of operation is apparent to users with little computer experience. Hard copy is generated at the moment of data entry and can then be signed in the manner of a normal prescription. This overcomes the potential medico-legal problems inherent in computer-based prescribing.

The disadvantages of this system are technical. The current unit is too heavy at 2.6 kg for easy portability. Similarly the present internal software is written in a non-standard language-making programming, is time-consuming and the operations which can be performed are of a limited range.

The unit is limited in the range of data which can be entered. For TPN prescribing it is ideal because the range of components is small. This is not the case for the majority of drug prescriptions although the ability to confine prescriptions to a defined choice of drugs might be of benefit for cost containment. In areas where a small range of prescribed drugs is used, such as in anaesthesia, this structured approach is applicable. This would be especially true for record keeping of chemotherapy protocols. More generally it is clear that much of the data input in medicine can be structured. Examples include follow-up at diabetic clinics, risk scoring and differential diagnosis of chest or abdominal pain where data capture systems using the pad could be easily implemented.

It is unlikely that paper will ever be entirely replaced in the medical environment. This approach to data entry, by mimicking the normal working practice attempts to fit the solution to the problem rather than vice-versa. A pad of this type, the size and weight of a clipboard, with easy programming, would have widespread application in medicine. If the portable pen on paper approach could be combined with recognition of characters and numeric values the problems of marrying the paper record with computer data entry will be overcome.

Further Reading

Clemmer TP, Larsen KG, Orme JF (1986) Computer applications in clinical nutrition. In: Rombeau JL, Caldwell MD (eds) Parenteral nutrition. W.B. Saunders, Philadelphia, pp 344–357 (Clinical Nutrition, vol 2)
Collinson PO, Jones RG (1987) Microcomputer applications in nutrition. In: Grant A, Todd E (eds) Enteral and parenteral nutrition, 2nd ed. Blackwell Scientific Publications, London, pp 109–112

10 A Critical Review of the Development of a Software Package for Clinical Urodynamics

J. G. Malone-Lee and C. R. Chapple

Introduction

Urodynamic investigation has undoubtedly been greatly refined and facilitated by the use of the modern generation of microcomputers which increase our ability to generate large quantities of physiological data. Manual techniques of data storage, analysis and interpretation are tedious, time-consuming and lead to observer transcription errors. The solution is to develop a software package to provide these facilities. A comprehensive data-processing system should fulfil the following criteria. It should be:

1. Easy to use and demand minimal computing experience
2. Fully interactive allowing for flexible storage, display, review and correction of data
3. Capable of incorporating comprehensive graphics options
4. Adaptable to individual requirements
5. Labour saving, with the collation of clinical information and urodynamic data into a standard report format
6. Run on cheap, readily available hardware

Urodynamics is a relatively new science which developed from work in California and Sweden in the 1950s and early 1960s (Miller 1979). It was subsequently refined into an important clinical investigative technique at the Middlesex Hospital in the late 1960s (Bates et al. 1970). Urodynamic investigation encompasses a number of techniques and assesses the functions of storage and voiding of urine by the bladder. The simplest techniques measure urinary flow rates and, using ultrasound or radiographic imaging, allow assessment of post-voiding bladder residuals. More complex clinical problems necessitate the measurement of filling pressure and then synchronous measurement of voiding pressures and flow rates (simple cystometry). The most accurate and complex procedure involves the additional radiographic screening of the patient (video-

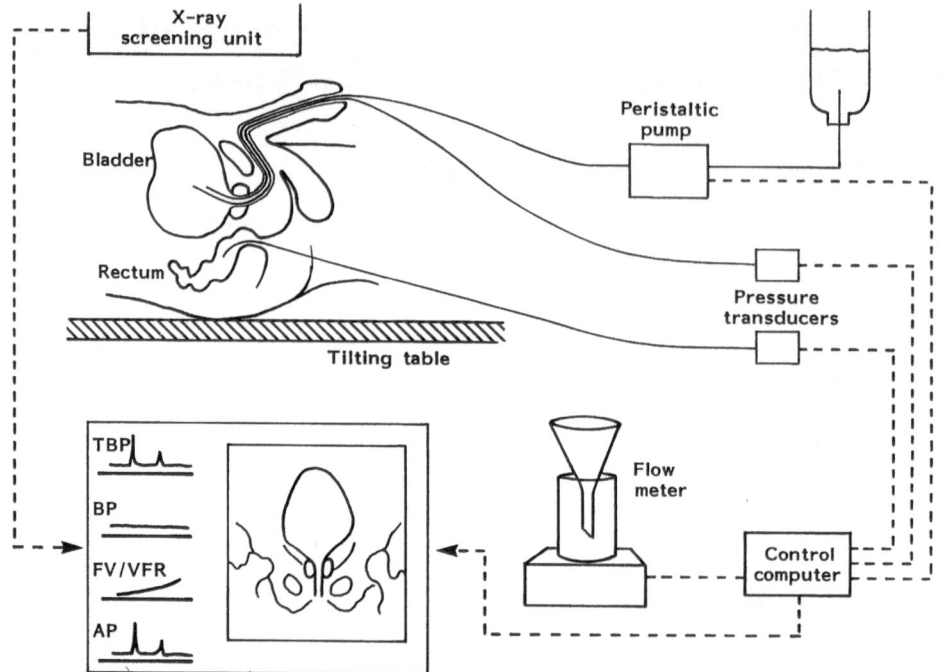

Fig. 10.1. Diagrammatic representation of the equipment required to perform simultaneous simple cystometry and cystourethrography. The bladder is filled at a predetermined rate with a radio-opaque contrast medium with the simultaneous measurement of bladder pressure (TBP) and rectal pressure (AP). The true detrusor pressure (BP) is calculated automatically (TBP−AP). Infused volume (FV) and the voiding flow rate (VFR) are recorded. This information with accompanying radiographic pictures and a sound track is recorded on video tape, allowing for subsequent review and analysis.

cystometry) and allows assessment of sphincteric action or the demonstration of anatomical abnormalities (Fig. 10.1).

A microcomputer is capable of collecting these data, analysing the information, producing reports and storing the data for subsequent retrieval. However, if the system is to be effective it must be sufficiently versatile to tolerate a wide variety of operators possessing different degrees of computer literacy. In addition, because a clinical history is an integral part of these investigations, user-friendly interaction via a keyboard must be a component of the system. This chapter describes our experiences in the development of a software package to aid clinicians performing urodynamic investigations.

The Selection of the Microcomputer

At the beginning of this project we decided that in order to maximise the speed and portability of the package the software would have to be designed for IBM-compatible machines. However, during the development of the software and before the efficacy of the project had been established we decided to work with a less expensive alternative. In 1983, the Acorn BBC microcomputer was selected as the machine for this project for the following reasons:

1. The low cost and ready availability of the microcomputer
2. The fact that it had a four-channel analogue port with an analogue to digital converter
3. The BBC microcomputer had excellent high resolution graphics facilities well-suited to urodynamic reporting
4. The Acorn BBC BASIC language was a well developed high level language that was versatile and relatively easy to master. It was possible to write structured programs suited to subsequent translation. It facilitated rapid alteration of software with minimal disruption

In 1986 the software package was redeveloped for the newer Acorn BBC Master Series microcomputer. This enabled the package to keep abreast of the substantial developments made by Acorn and to take advantage of the 64 K of memory available on this machine. The current package runs on a BBC Master Series Microcomputer with a four drive 80 track disc, a high resolution colour monitor and an Epson FX series printer. The interface between microcomputer and urodynamic equipment ensures that the maximum signal applied to the computer analogue input does not exceed 1.8 volts. Hard copies of texts are produced by standard alphanumeric printing, and graphics are reproduced by an Epson specific graphics screen dump.

The Selection of a Programmer

In the early stages of the project we intended that a physicist would write the programs. Limited resources made it impossible to employ a person who would be available for the considerable time required to become familiar with all aspects of the urodynamic investigation. This resulted in early programs being unsuitable for the clinicians operating the microcomputers. It was decided that a physician running a urodynamic department should learn to program and then develop a customised system. It took 18 months for the first author (JML) to gain the competence in programming needed to achieve the results that were planned. It took 4 years to produce the current system.

Product Development

In the early stages of development we discovered that it was unwise for the programmer to test the acceptability of the software until it had been tried by other people who were inexperienced with computers and were working unsupervised by the programmer. The writer could sense problems in his own software and manipulate the system so as to circumvent difficulties. Other users could not do this and precipitated failures of the system.

The package was first used in the programmer's own department where he supervised four nurses and one doctor over 12 months. The software was continually altered in response to failures in this environment. The system was then established in the Urodynamic Department of the Royal National Orthopaedic Hospital and the same process repeated but with the programmer off-site while the software was being used. Further problems were encountered and solved as a result of this trial. The final off-site validation was carried out in the Urodynamic Department at the Middlesex Hospital. This resulted in radical changes in the whole structure of the package, expanding facilities for history collection and the incorporation of radiographic details.

As well as being an excellent way of discovering bugs in the system, the process of off-site unsupervised validation helped to enrich the software. Different units had different styles and therefore made novel demands of the programmer. All of the departments involved in this project had to endure long weeks of frustrating and exasperating breakdowns in the system. We learnt that it was essential for the programmer to be punctilious about accepting responsibility for failure and altering his software to accommodate operator aberrations. There was nothing to be gained from blaming an operator as new personnel made the same errors. The computer had to be taught to think around the operator and not vice versa.

The Final Product

At the end of the trials the software package development on the BBC machines was concluded. The current system consists of 15 programs and these are to be adapted for use on an IBM-compatible machine using the "C" programming language. These programs link into each other, one calling up the next in sequence. A series of menus aid the operator in selecting the various options available. These programs are:

1. The initialisation program which demands a password before moving on to the next in sequence
2. The main system menu which permits access to the various facilities available
3. The entry of a new patient's details, including the clinical history. This program selects a number for the patient and reserves storage space for the patient's file
4. The urodynamic study program. This collects all the analogue data displaying the pressure and flow parameters on an easily readable bar chart. It has facilities for marking events. The pressure readings can be balanced and there are scaling facilities for unusually large values. Pause facilities allow the study to be interrupted if necessary

5. Supplementary data program, which accepts data such as radiographic findings, entered by the operator. It then proceeds to collate the urodynamic data and calculate the main reporting variables such as end filling pressure etc.

6. Main patient recall facility. This program loads the entire urodynamic study into the computer. By means of a sequence of menus it permits reporting of parameters and graphics in a wide variety of ways. Hard copy of any screen can be obtained

7. Patient clinical history and report program, which will provide hard copy on request

8. Edit facility to permit correction of any erroneous entries in the patient's file

9. Standard non-graphic urodynamic report and clinical history printing program

10. Standard urodynamic report program with graphics for one or more patients. It is used for producing batches of reports at the end of a clinic

11. Urodynamic report program with the filling study graphics and voiding study graphics produced separately on four channels. This provides data on one or more patients

12. Report and clinical history program for one or more patients but without any graphics records

13. Program to locate a named patient's file or files using an index

14, 15. These programs are custom designed to use for recall of patient data during weekly review meetings. A number of departments have these meetings and a customised recall facility is very useful

The fifteen programs that make up the software package are stored on the "0" drive surface of a 400-kbyte 80-track disc. A 200-kbyte index of patients is stored on the "2" drive surface of the 80 track disc used for the programs. The index can hold 3000 patient names. A 400-kbyte 80-track disc uses the "1" and "3" drive surfaces to store individual patient files. Each of these discs can hold 28 patient files. Each patient is allocated 14 kbytes of disc memory.

At the start of a urodynamic study the microcomputer accesses the storage disc and allocates 14 kbytes of space. If there is no room, the operator is instructed to change to a new disc. The patient's record file is a random access file. The first 300 bytes are used to store clinical history details (58 individual alphanumeric entries). The next 300 bytes are used to store the main urodynamic parameters (37 individual integer entries). The remainder of the space is used to store the abdominal pressure, bladder pressure and flow rate parameters which are sampled every second and immediately written to disc. There is enough space for a 17-minute test. All numeric variables are stored as integers. During the urodynamic study the variables recorded are not stored in the microcomputer but are written to disc. This protects the data against program corruption. The times of important events in the study, which cannot be written immediately to disc, are stored as resident integer variables which will survive any problem short of a power failure. The break key is programmed to resuscitate the study data in the event of an operator-induced failure. A patient's file is also protected against accidental overwriting. These facilities have proven successful in protecting the data collected from serious errors.

Some of the Lessons Learned

The programs contained errors which had to be gradually weeded out by the programmer. It took a long time to discover all of the programming bugs. The last known one was discovered after 9 months of successful operation. A more important source of error came from the operators themselves. We found that users were quick to report disastrous failures but often ignored or failed to recognise less conspicuous problems. These could be detected by viewing the patients' files from time to time and by watching the operators using the equipment. We found it important for the programmer to avoid the temptation to offer advice on operation techniques when he was present at a urodynamic study. A more lasting solution was to instruct the microcomputer to respond intelligently to variations in operator style. We found it remarkable that users proved surprisingly tolerant of obvious inefficiencies in the system and frequently failed to notice improvements that had been worked in. The main source of operator error was the entry of meaningless data. We found it safer to get the computer to suggest a file number for a patient and to always default to this number unless otherwise instructed. All numeric entries needed to be checked by the microcomputer for quality and erroneous entries rejected. A common error was the entry of "O" (letter) instead "0" (number) for zero, or "I" instead of "1" for one. The entry of the clinicial history made greatest demands on programming. Because of the limitations of space most computer systems guide the entry of data by means of preselected options. For instance, the response to a question may require a "Y" or "N" and nothing else. You can also use numeric scales such as "1 = never, 2 = occasional, 3 = usual". Though this approach is helpful, it is also restricting. We found that it was possible to adapt the process so that although preselected options were used the operator could, if necessary, qualify a response by typing in a short statement such as "very rarely". The microcomputer was programmed to search the answers to detect such entries and reproduce them when they occurred. This option was much appreciated by the operators. The memory allocation proved ample for this type of approach.

Problems were encountered over variations in the use of upper and lower-case characters. We found that this was solved by arranging to convert all data entries automatically to a standard format. Because typing entries were an important source of error we found it necessary to provide copious error-correction facilities which served to reassure the operators. With these provisos we did not encounter difficulties as a result of keyboard data entry. We noted that operators frequently became lost within the program sequence and the microcomputer had to remind users where they were. The use of sound and colour proved invaluable as subliminal prompts to operators. A booting facility enabled the operators to return to the main program menu at any stage and standardised escape facilities always returned the operator to the beginning of a particular program. A more serious problem was created when a careless operator accidentally pressed a wrong key during the urodynamic study. We found that many disasters could be avoided by disabling redundant keys and by programming the powerful break key to link back into the recording programs without losing data. We also found that it was possible to program the computer to make sensible decisions if data entry was incomplete. These facilities combined with the approach to storage rendered the data gathering procedures surprisingly resilient to human error.

We discovered that people found it difficult to wait while data were being loaded or plotted. This often resulted in impatient tapping of the keys. Though this practice caused no harm to the running of the system operators clearly found it disquieting. Requests for patience and the use of sound to signal the end of loading and plotting procedures eased this difficulty. "Chatty" comments from the microcomputer, though endearing, only served to persuade the operators that the machine was more intelligent that it was. Many operators had expectations of judgement by the machine that could be fulfilled because the investigation takes place according to a defined protocol.

Conclusion

This system has now been running successfully in three urodynamic departments for more than twelve months without problems, despite the fact that the operators are constantly changing. We believe that it is possible to design packages for clinical use that incorporate keyboard interaction provided that carefully validated error-trapping facilities are included within the programs.

References

Bates CP, Whiteside G, Turner Warwick RT (1970) Synchronous cine/pressure/flow cysto-urethro-graphy with special reference to stress and urge incontinence. Br J Urol 42: 714–723
Miller E (1979) The Beginnings. Symposium on Clinic Urodynamics. Urol Clin N Am 6: 7–9

11 A Study of the Validity of Voiding Pressure – Flow Plot Interpretation in Clinical Urodynamics

C. R. Chapple and J. G. Malone-Lee

Introduction

The principles of urodynamic investigation and our approach to them using microcomputer technology have been described in the previous chapter. This paper describes a specific application of our technique to diagnosis. Although many departments have access to simple urodynamic procedures there are a number of situations where it is not possible, without the use of more complex investigations such as videocystometry, to exclude outflow obstruction or to clarify the pathology. In addition, the successful interpretation of urodynamic data is largely subjective and dependent on the investigator's experience. We have studied an alternative method of diagnosing the presence of lower urinary tract obstruction from urodynamic traces, made possible by microcomputers, which is easier to use because it depends on "pattern recognition". The human brain may be more efficient at interpreting the meaning of patterns than it is at interpreting numeric data. Microcomputers enable us to plot the analogue data obtained from urodynamic studies in a variety of different ways. We have used a microcomputer system, described in the previous chapter, to generate specific plots which have very characteristic patterns depending on the pathological circumstances.

This chapter is based on the work published by Griffiths (1973, 1977, 1980) who described the principle of plotting the detrusor pressure against the flow rate during micturition. The resultant curve has a pattern, the shape of which is influenced by the urethral resistance relationship (URR) and its position by the bladder output relationship (BOR). This technique involves a re-structuring of data readily available from standard urodynamic studies which already reflect the curves. Early experience with plotting these curves using a microcomputer suggested that urodynamic diagnosis could be aided by recognition of characteristic "patterns" suggesting particular pathologies, especially where the findings

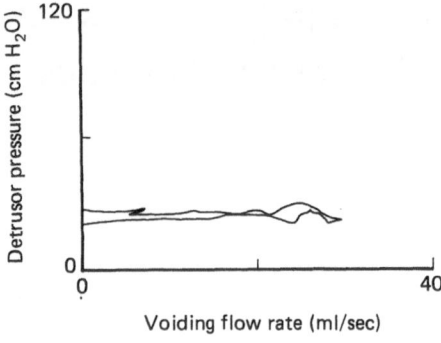

Fig. 11.1. A plot from an unobstructed urethra.

were equivocal. Examination of the curves is fascinating and it is tempting to read much into what they express. Because of this we decided to submit their use to a simple but stark experiment. Our aim was to compare pure interpretation of the plots, in the absence of any supplementary information, with the results of formal video-urodynamic investigation.

Method

A double blind study was designed. Urodynamic data were collected during video-urodynamic studies conducted at the Middlesex Hospital with the equipment described in other presentations (Malone-Lee 1987; Chapple et al. 1987) It should be noted that the data were sampled at 1 Hertz. The plots of pressure against flow were examined and classified by one observer (JML) who was given no other information. No attempt was made to calculate the estimated maximum urinary flow (Griffiths 1977) on the BOR because of doubts concerning the validity of the isometric pressure during voluntary inhibition of micturition. The written video-urodynamic study reports were collated by another observer (CRC) who was unaware of the pressure against flow plot classifications or how they were being interpreted. The findings of the two observers were then compared.

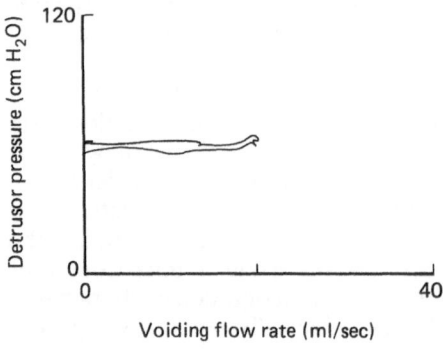

Fig. 11.2. A plot from an unobstructed urethra.

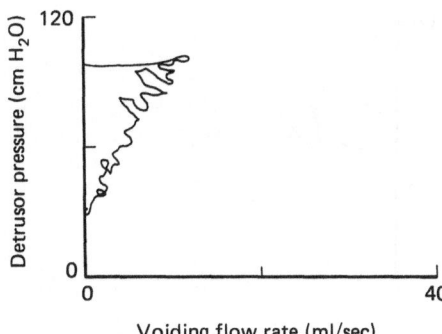

Fig. 11.3. A plot from an obstructed urethra.

Results

Four hundred and twenty three studies were analysed. Of these 110 failed to produce proper voiding studies either because the patient failed to void or because of technical problems: 313 voiding pressure against flow plots were examined.

Plots which were thought by the observer (JML) to reflect an unobstructed and distensible urethra were classified into two groups. Samples of the types of plot are shown in Figs. 11.1, 11.2. Like all of the samples shown these should not be considered to give exhaustive representation. Ninety three patients were classified into these two groups, 73 women and 20 men. Their mean age was 51 yr (±15), their mean bladder capacity was 477 ml (±178) and their mean voided volume was 444 ml (±153). The video-urodynamic reports described 85 (91%) of these patients as unobstructed. Eight patients (9%) were reported as being obstructed and only one of these was a male. The seven women were reported as "mildly" or "possibly" obstructed.

Three classes of pattern were selected as suggesting some form of obstruction with parts of the traces approaching the behaviour of rigid tubes. These are shown in Figs. 11.3, 11.4 and 11.5. Ninety patients fell into these categories, 22 women and 68 men. Their mean age was 58 yr (±15), their mean bladder capacity was 433 ml (±153) and their mean voided volume was 359 ml (±152). Of these patients,

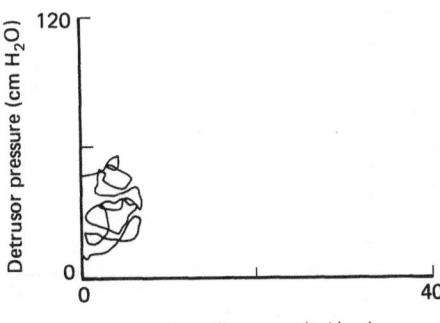

Fig. 11.4. A plot from an obstructed urethra.

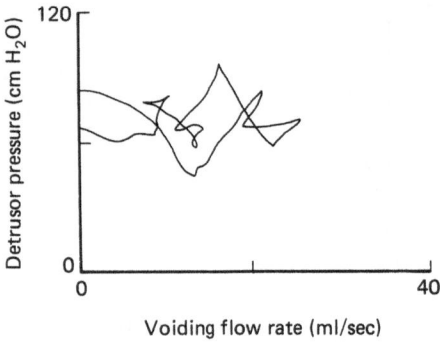

Fig. 11.5. A plot from an obstructed urethra. Obstruction due to urethral kinking from bladder base descent.

79 (88%) were reported as demonstrating evidence of obstruction on video-urodynamic investigation. Of the 11 patients who were reported as showing no evidence of obstruction the first author had expressed reservations about his choice of classification of 9 prior to comparison of the findings.

Thirty-one patients were classified into two groups (Figs. 11.6, 11.7) which suggested an underactive detrusor. This was naive and not up to the experimental design as many of these studies were technically faulted and the second author was not aware of this. In only 45% of these studies was an underactive detrusor considered to be the principal urodynamic diagnosis.

The 99 other patients produced plots that were difficult to classify. Many of these (64) were found to have a low capacity detrusor instability with a low volume void. A number of others were rejected because it was found that their plots resulted from faulted studies because of early problems with the equipment.

Discussion

Though these plots were interpreted without any supplementary data, which would not be the case in normal practice, it is encouraging to note considerable agreement with formal video-urodynamic investigation. With the development of

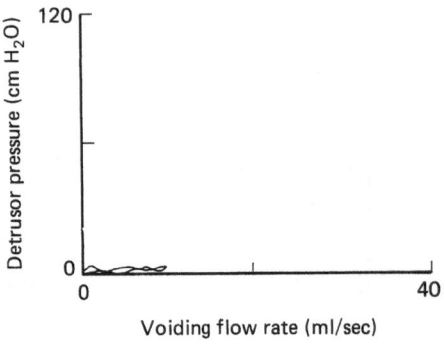

Fig. 11.6. A plot thought to be due to detrusor underactivity.

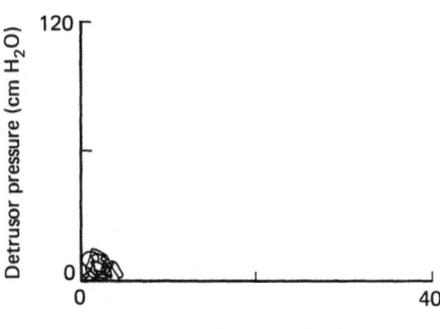

Fig. 11.7. A plot thought to be due to
detrusor underactivity.

microcomputers this technique should become more readily available and our
skill in interpretation should grow. The main advantage of these plots is that they
concisely depict the whole of the voiding phase and thereby avoid errors incurred
by giving exclusive emphasis to the maximum flow rate and accompanying
detrusor pressure (Abrams and Griffiths 1979). It also appears that interpretation
can be valid using "pattern" recognition. It is likely that this technique will be of
greatest value where more sophisticated facilities are not readily available. What
is certain is that much more discussion and awareness of this approach is
warranted.

References

Abrams PH, Griffiths DJ (1979) The assessment of prostatic obstruction from urodynamic
    measurements and from residual urine. Br J Urol 51: 129–134
Chapple CR, Malone-Lee JG, Rickards D, Milroy EJG, Turner Warwick RT (1987) A comprehen-
    sive microcomputer software package for videocystometry, Neurol Urodynam 6: 208–209
Griffiths DJ (1973) The mechanics of the urethra and of micturition. Br J Urol 45: 497–507
Griffiths DJ (1977) Urodynamic assessment of bladder function. Br J Urol 49: 29–36
Griffiths DJ (1980) Urodynamics: the mechanics and hydrodynamics of the lower urinary tract. Adam
    Hilger, Bristol
Malone-Lee JG (1987) Experience in software development for a microcomputer in clinical
    urodynamics. Neurol Urodynam 6: 200–201

12 Left Ventricular Volume and Valve Gradient Analysis using an Apple Macintosh Computer

S.W. Hughes, I.C. Cooper, D. Katritsis and M.M. Webb-Peploe

Introduction

Two programs, MacAngio and MacValve, have been developed to automate the analysis of cardiac catheterisation data.

Hardware

The programs run on any of the Macintosh family of computers connected to a suitable digitising tablet, such as the MacTablet (Summagraphics Corp., Connecticut). The equipment is shown in Fig. 12.1. The programs have been written and compiled in Zbasic (Zedcor Inc., Tucson, Arizona). Zbasic enables programs to use the Macintosh user interface routines. The Mac interface is often referred to by the acronym WIMP, which stands for windows, icons, mouse and pointers. These features make the Macintosh family of computers exceptionally easy to use.

MacAngio

Introduction

Cardiac cine-angiography has been used for the measurement of left ventricular (LV) chamber volume for more than 30 years. In this procedure, a catheter is inserted through the aortic valve into the LV. As radio-opaque contrast media is injected via the catheter into the ventricle 35-mm cine X-ray pictures are taken (Fig. 12.1).

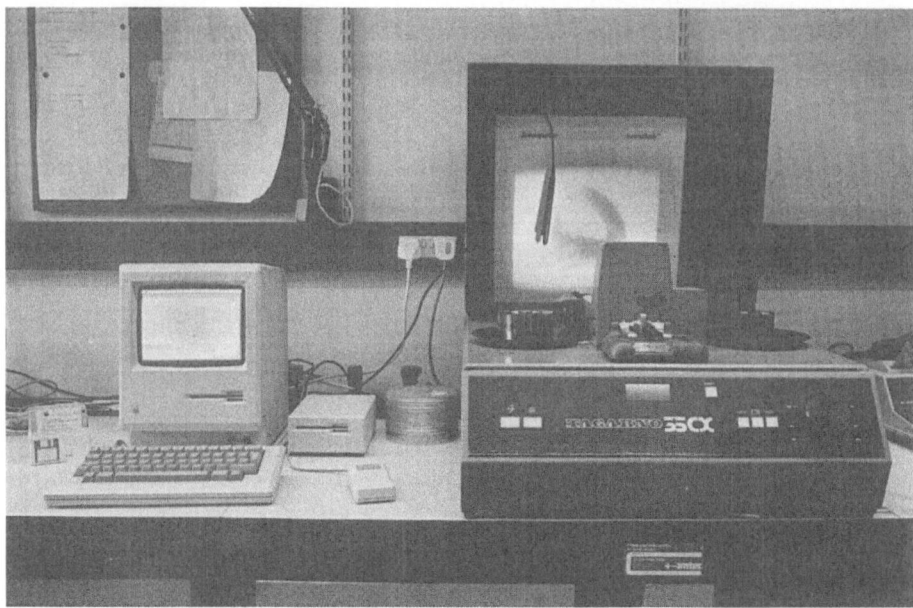

Fig. 12.1. The Macintosh computer system and the cine angiogram projector. An image of a left ventricle in end diastole is seen projected onto the digitising tablet. The tracing stylus is seen hanging down in front of the tablet. Wall motion radials are seen on the screen of the Macintosh computer.

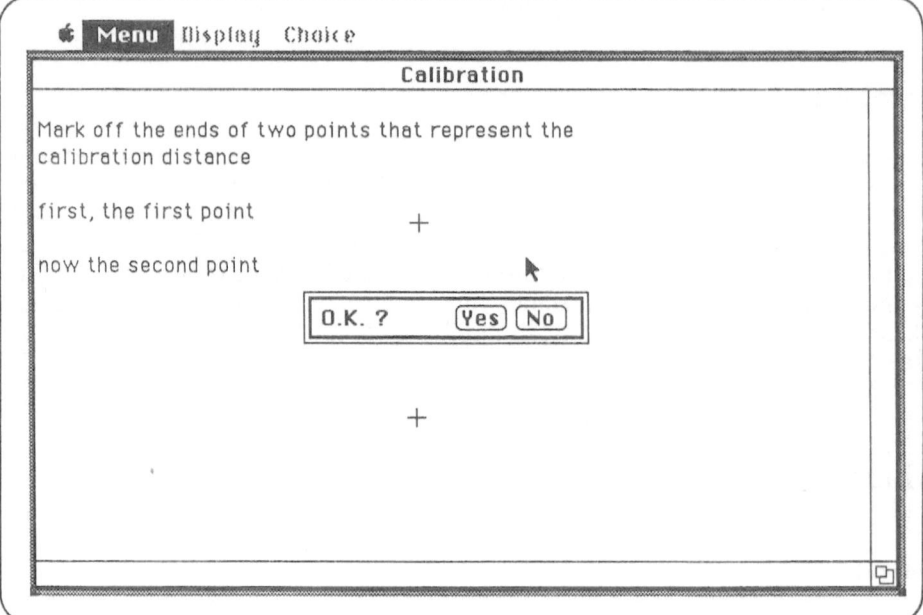

Fig. 12.2. Screen display showing a dialogue box. An outline which has just been traced may be either accepted or rejected.

Software

Before running MacAngio, the digitising tablet is switched on using the Apple menu which appears in the top left corner of the screen (Fig. 12.2). The active area of the tablet is mapped onto the computer screen. When the stylus is moved across the surface a pointer moves across the computer screen (seen in Fig. 12.2). The active area of the tablet may be changed. Changing the active area changes the digitising resolution. Normally the active area is set to about 27×27 cm, giving a resolution of about 0.6 mm, which is adequate for digitising LV outlines.

On double-clicking the MacAngio icon, a menu bar labelled Menu appears at the top left of the screen. When the pointer is moved onto the menu bar and the mouse button pressed, a pull-down menu appears on the screen. MacAngio comprises five modules which are run from this main menu:

Main menu
1. Trace outline
2. Analyse outlines
3. Display results
4. Trace-analyse-print
5. Quick ejection fraction
6. Finish

Trace Outline

Before tracing the outlines, an information form must be filled in. The following information is required.

1. Catheter number
2. Date (default today's date)
3. Name of patient
4. Hospital number
5. Date of birth
6. Body surface area (m^2)
7. Calibration distance (default 6 cm)
8. Frame rate (default 50 Hz)
9. No. of frames between the ED and ES frames

Calibration. A calibration distance (usually 6 cm) is recorded on the cine film by moving the table on which the patient is lying a set distance while the catheter is in the ventricle. The calibration reference points are transferred to the computer by marking the points with the stylus held over the projected X-ray image.

Tracing. End systolic (ES) and end diastolic (ED) LV outlines are traced (Fig. 12.1). Up to 395 points are allowed in each outline. The outlines must be oriented with the valve plane at the top left and the apex at the bottom right. Each outline tracing is started at the top of the valve plane and ended at the bottom of the valve plane. A double click on the mouse indicates that the outline has been finished. An "O.K. Yes/No?" dialogue box appears on the screen. If a mistake has been made the tracing may be repeated by clicking on the "No" box. A section of wall may be traced if a wall mass calculation is required.

If wall mass is required, two lines, about 1–2 cm long, are traced along the outer and inner section of the wall. The mean thickness is calculated by dividing the area of the section by the mean length of the two lines. When all the tracings have been completed the data are stored on disc. A file name is constructed from the angio number, date and name of the patient, e.g.:

angio 1 88 A Patient

Analysis

The analysis module inputs the trace data from the disc, analyses the data, and stores the results on disc. Storage and retrieval of data on the disc is made very easy by the user interface. A dialogue box appears on the screen listing the angio files on the currently selected disc. A file is selected by double clicking on the filename. The analysis module is in two parts: volume analysis and wall motion analysis.

Volume analysis. Chamber volumes are calculated by two methods, the Dodge method and the multi-slice method (Yang et al. 1978). In the Dodge method, the chamber is assumed to be an ellipsoid of revolution, i.e. the volume described by an ellipse rotated 360° about the major axis. To calculate the volume of an ellipsoid of revolution, the lengths of the major and minor axes must be known. The long axis is defined (in MacAngio) as a line running from the mid-point of the valve plane to the apex. The apex is defined as the point on the outline furthest away from the mid-point of the valve plane. The length of the minor axis of an ellipse with an area equivalent to that of the chamber outline is found by dividing the area of the outline by the length of the major axis. The volume of an ellipsoid of revolution is given by:

$$V = \frac{\pi\, a^2 b}{6}$$

where a is the major axis and b is the minor axis.

The Dodge volume is calculated for the ED and ES frames. An empirical correction is applied to the single plane volumes to bring them into line with biplane values:

$$Vol_b = 0.81\ Vol_s + 1.9\ ml$$

Multi-slice Method. This method divides each outline into a number of slices that run perpendicular to the long axis (Fig. 12.3). Each slice is assumed to be a disc. The volume of each disc is found by multiplying the area by the thickness. The total chamber volume is found by adding up all the disc volumes. The number of slices to be used in the multi-slice model may be specified before analysis and may be varied from 3 to 50 (default 10).

The Dodge and multi-slice volumes are used to calculate the following:

End diastolic volume (EDV)
End systolic volume (ESV)

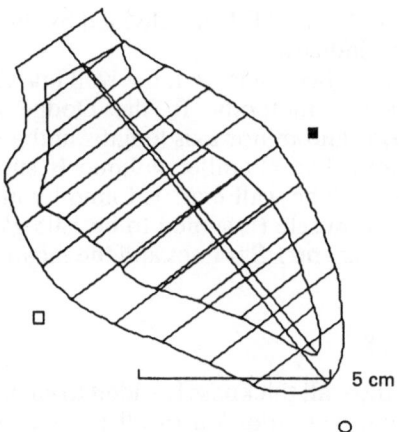

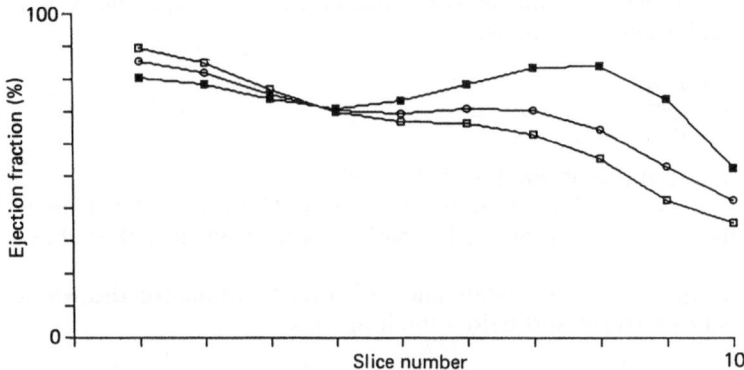

Fig. 12.3. Slice ejection fractions. The top diagram shows two (ED and ES) outlines divided up into 10 slices. The graph shows the ejection fraction for each slice and for the slice sections above and below the long axes. The solid squares correspond to the ejection fractions calculated for the sections above the long axis, and the open squares for those below. The open circles correspond to the ejection fractions calculated for the whole slice.

Stroke volume (SV)
Ejection fraction (EJFR)
Ejection rate (ER)
Normalised ejection rate (NER)
SV = EDV − ESV
EJFR = SV/EDV
ER = SV/ET
NER = EJFR × ET

(ET is the ejection time in seconds)

All of these values, except EJFR and ET, are divided by the body surface area (in square metres) to produce indices.

If the wall thickness option has been selected, the wall mass is calculated using both the Dodge and multi-slice methods. In the Dodge method, the wall thickness is added to the major and minor axis lengths and a volume calculated for the ellipsoid of revolution. The chamber volume is subtracted from this volume to give the wall volume. The wall mass is found by multiplying the wall volume by the density of heart muscle (assumed to be 1.05 g/cm in MacAngio). The mass is calculated for the ED and ES frames and the mean taken. The mass is biplane corrected:

$$\text{Mass}_b = 0.9 \, \text{Mass}_s + 15 \text{ g}$$

In the multi-slice method, the wall thickness is added to each slice diameter and a new disc volume calculated. The addition of all the disc volumes gives the chamber volume plus the wall volume. The multi-slice chamber volume is subtracted from the chamber volume plus wall volume to give the wall volume. The wall mass is calculated by multiplying the wall volume by the density of heart muscle.

The shape index for each outline is also calculated. The shape index is a measure of how circular each outline is.

$$\text{shape index} = \frac{4 \pi A}{p^2}$$

where A is the area and p the perimeter of the outline.

The shape index of a circle is 1 and that of a line is zero. Generally, the shape of an ED outline is more rounded than an ES outline and so has a higher shape index.

The slice volumes are used to calculate slice ejection fractions for the whole slice and for the sections above and below the long axis.

Wall motion. The analysis of heart wall motion enables a quantitative assessment of heart function. The slice diameters are used to calculate transverse wall motion for each diameter and for each of the sections above and below the long axis.

$$\text{Wall}_t = \frac{(L_{ed} - L_{es}) \times 100}{L_{ed}}$$

The slice diameters are also used to calculate circumferential velocity of fibre shortening (vcf) at each diameter and above and below the long axis.

$$\text{vcf} = \frac{C_{ed} - C_{es}}{C_{ed} - ET}$$

where C is the circumference (cm) and ET the ejection time in seconds.

Radial wall motion is also calculated. Firstly, a centre of strain is calculated for the ED and ES outlines. The centre of strain (CST) is a point on the long axis that most of the points on the outline tend to be moving towards as the heart contracts. This is normally taken as a point 69% down the long axis going from the valve plane to the apex of the heart. In MacAngio the CST may be varied between 0 and 100%, but in practice would normally be either 69% or 50%. The ES outline is translated so that its CST overlays that of the ED outline. The long axis of the ES frame is then rotated so that it lies over the long axis of the ED frame. The two outlines are divided into a number of segments (default 12) centred on the CST (Fig. 12.3). The contraction is calculated at each radial.

$$\text{Wall}_r = \frac{R_{ed} - R_{es} \times 100}{R_{ed}}$$

The results are saved in the same file as the outline data.

Display

The display nodule recalls and displays the outline data and the results of the analysis. The display menu has three options: Summary report, walkthrough, choice. The summary report prints out the patient details, volume analysis, and the wall motion results (Figs. 12.4, 12.5). Walkthrough displays all of the result pages in turn. Choice enables individual pages to be displayed and printed out as required.

Quick Ejection Fraction

This module enables the quick calculation of EDV, ESV, SV, EJFR and their indices (the first three values divided by body surface area in metres). The outlines and the results may be printed out.

MacValve

Introduction

MacValve is a program used for measuring valve gradients. For example, the mean pressure gradient between the left atrium (LA) and left ventricle (LV) is used to diagnose and assess the degree of mitral stenosis. Likewise the mean pressure gradient between the LV and the aorta assesses the degree of aortic stenosis. Intravascular pressure recordings obtained from patients undergoing cardiac catheterisation are used for analysis. When measuring valve gradients the simultaneous record of two chambers (e.g. LV and aorta) are required. These records may be placed on the digitising tablet. The tablet is put into high resolution mode (0.2 mm).

MacValve comprises four main modules: calibration, trace, cursors, printout.

Summary Angio Report

Name	test patient
Date of angio	28/05/87
Angio no.	2
Hospital no.	999
DoB	20-4-58
BSA	2

	Dodge	M.S.	Index Dodge	M.S.
end-diastolic volume	188	232.3	94	116.2
end-systolic volume	60.5	73.8	30.3	36.9
stroke volume (ml)	127.5	158.5	63.8	79.3
ejection rate	318.8	396.3	159.4	198.1
normalised ejection rate	127.5	158.5	63.8	79.3
ejection fraction	.68	.68		
wall mass (g)	0	0		
ejection time (s)	.4			

	ES	ED
long axis length	9.8	11.5
chamber area	28.9	55.8
wall thickness	0	0
shape index	.6	.76

Mean vcf = 1.01 cm/s

(N.B. Dodge volumes have been biplane corrected)

Fig. 12.4. The first page of an angio summary report.

Calibration

During the catheterisation procedure, time and pressure calibration marks are put onto the recording paper. The distances on the paper representing the calibration time (e.g. 1 second) and the pressure (e.g. 100 mm Hg) are marked off by using the digitising stylus.

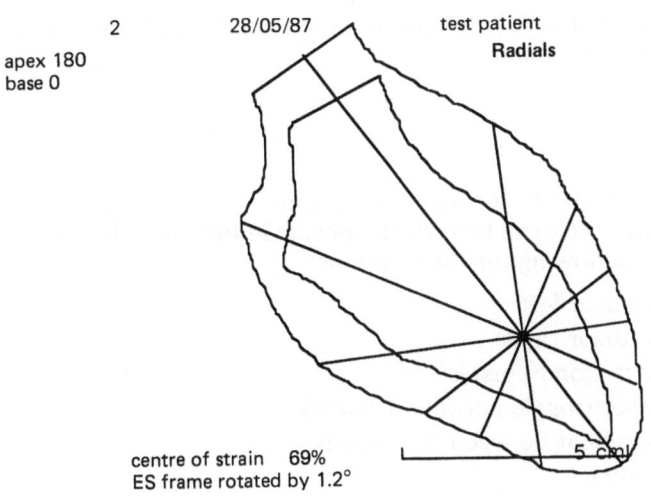

2   28/05/87   test patient
apex 180   Radials
base 0

centre of strain   69%
ES frame rotated by 1.2°

Radial contraction

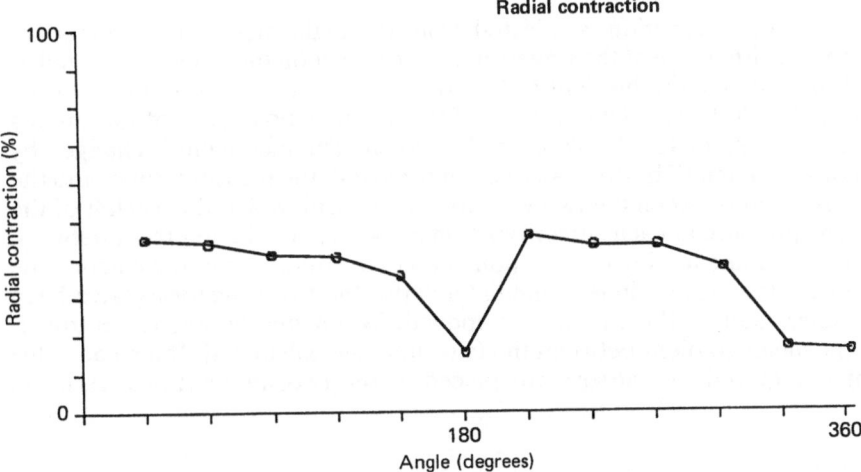

Fig. 12.5. The second page of an angio summary report. The top diagram shows two left ventricular outlines (ED and ES) with wall motion radials superimposed. The bottom diagram shows a plot of percentage radial contraction versus angle.

Trace

Before tracing the waveforms an origin is selected. This is the reference point for time and pressure. Normally the origin would be set at zero time and pressure but it may be set at any value of time and pressure. For instance the origin could be set at zero time and 20 mm Hg pressure, in which case 20 mm Hg would be added to subsequent pressure readings. After the origin has been marked, two pressure waveforms are traced by using the stylus. The waveforms appear on the computer screen as they are traced. Up to 200 points are allowed for each waveform. A trace is terminated by double clicking on the mouse button, and the trace is either accepted or rejected by clicking on a "Yes/No" dialogue box (as in MacAngio).

A rejected trace must be retraced. When both the waveforms have been traced the program returns to the main menu.

Cursors

Two cursors may be moved across the two superimposed waveforms. These cursors are controlled from a dialogue box which appears in the top right corner of the screen. This has the following function buttons:

Left: Move selected cursor left
Right: Move selected cursor right
1 <> 10:   Move the cursors 1 or 10 pixels
Cursor: Change the cursor (toggle between 1 and 2)
Gradient: Calculate the gradient between the cursors
Printout: Print-out the screen
Quit?   Return to the main menu

When the cursor function is selected from the main menu, two cursors are drawn, one on either side of the waveforms. The cursor on the left is designated as Cursor 1 and the one on the right as Cursor 2. These are moved left or right by clicking on the "left" or "right" button of the dialogue box. Each of the cursors may be moved one or ten divisions on the screen. The increment is changed by clicking on the "cursor" button. As a cursor is moved, the pressure, time, and the pressure gradient between the two waveforms are displayed at the top left of the screen. The pressure at each cursor position is found from the intercept between the cursor and a line joining the two points that fall either side of the cursor. The pressure calculations are done immediately after the two waveforms have been traced rather than as the cursors are moved. When the "gradient" button is clicked the mean gradient between the two cursors is calculated. If a mean valve gradient is required the cursors are placed at the two intersections. A mean

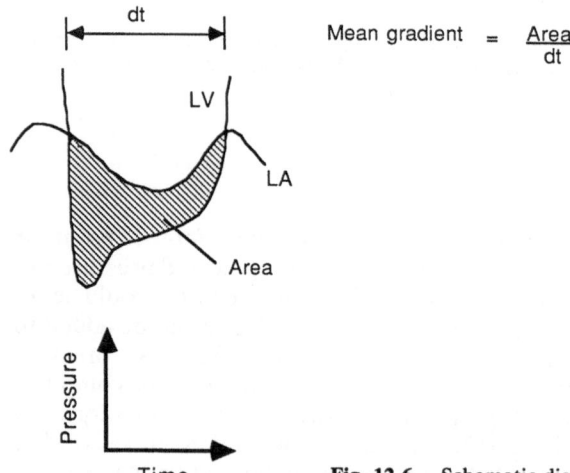

Fig. 12.6.   Schematic diagram of a LV–LA valve gradient.

gradient is calculated by first calculating the area under each curve between the cursors. The difference in area is divided by the time interval between the cursors (Fig. 12.6). This gives a mean height, which is multiplied by the pressure calibration factor to give the mean gradient. The maximum and minimum pressure gradient between the cursors is also calculated. The individual pressure values between the cursors are used to calculate the standard deviation of the mean gradient. After a gradient calculation the cursors may be re-positioned and a new calculation carried out if necessary.

Printout

A print-out of the screen may be obtained by clicking on the "printout" button.

References

Yang SS, Bentivoglio LG, Maranhão V, Goldberg H et al. (1978). From cardiac catheterisation data to haemodynamic parameters. F. A. Davis, Philadelphia

13 Computer-Assisted Bone-Marrow Reporting

O.H.B. Gyde

Introduction

Much of the steady and apparently inexhaustible increase in the workload of haematology laboratories has been met by automation and computerisation, without a corresponding increase in staff. However, routine accurate recognition and differentiation of all the blood and bone-marrow cells together with their many abnormal variants is beyond the current capability of computerised image processing and analysis and remains for the present a human activity. It is a labour-intensive task, particularly for the present-day haematologist who will often have an increasingly heavy clinical commitment.

Bone marrow contains a wide range of haemopoietic and supporting cells. When aspirated through a needle and spread on a glass slide the structural relationships are lost but the individual detail of cells is seen clearly. A biopsy taken with a wider bore needle and sectioned will show less of single cells but will demonstrate the anatomical arrangement. Both types of sample present the trainee haematologist with large numbers of cells of differing maturity and lineage that have to be identified and quantified. Computers should facilitate the work of the haematologist by allowing direct entry of his findings and the generation of reports. In addition, the less experienced will receive instruction by following the same protocol requiring the identification and enumeration of the cells in an orderly sequence. These data form the basis for subsequent interpretation and conclusions. Further help in the form of image processing allows easier counting, and measurement of cell shape and content. Automated advice from the computer may take the form of logical conclusions that can be drawn from the descriptions, or recorded photographic examples of cell types may be shown for comparison.

The Computer System

The original system was a BBC model B with a "Termi" communications chip allowing VT100 emulation and access to the main laboratory computer for the

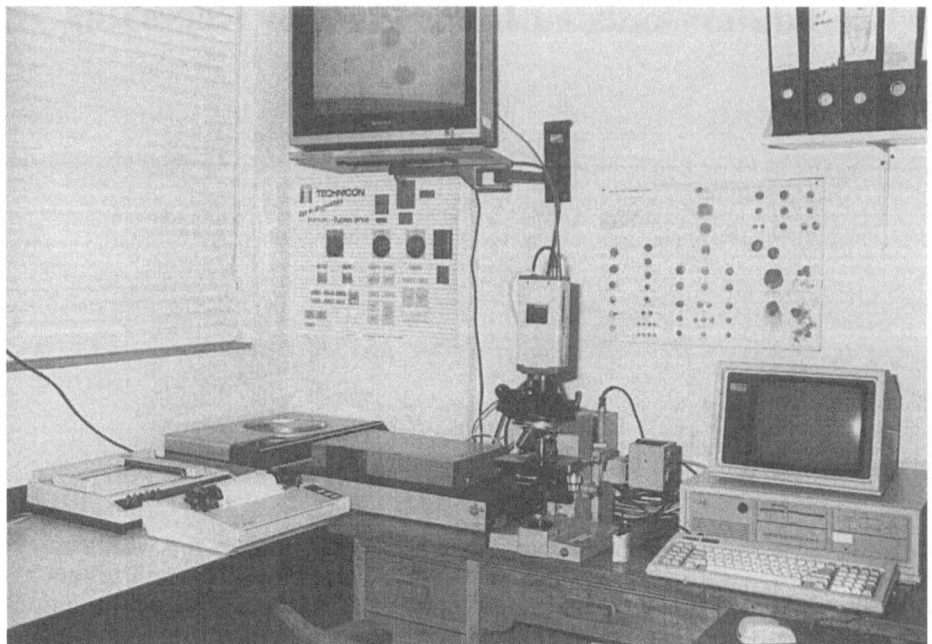

Fig. 13.1. General layout of the equipment.

reporting program. A counting program written in BBC BASIC was added (Clarke et al. 1985). It was impossible to run image analysis or expert systems of any complexity on this computer. The next stage required a Research Machines Nimbus X10, 8086 based microprocessor. At the present time, in order to achieve the IBM compatibility necessary to run the current programs at a reasonable speed, a Compaq Deskpro 286 is used.

The Compaq is used alongside the microscope in our laboratory to form a nucleus and to allow development of assisted reporting (Fig. 13.1). Switching on the computer boots up a menu of all the programs in the order that they are commonly used. Selection is made directly from the keyboard or by a mouse.

A direct link to the main haematology laboratory computer (a DEC 11/84 processor) is extremely helpful in providing a rapid check of the clinical details and the results of relevant blood tests (Fig. 13.2). Software emulation of a DEC VT100 visual display unit by the microprocessor converts it into a peripheral terminal giving instant access to all the laboratory information.

Marrow Reporting Software

The marrow aspirate or biopsy reporting program consists of a sequence of screens, each containing a set of questions about a cell type. These cover number,

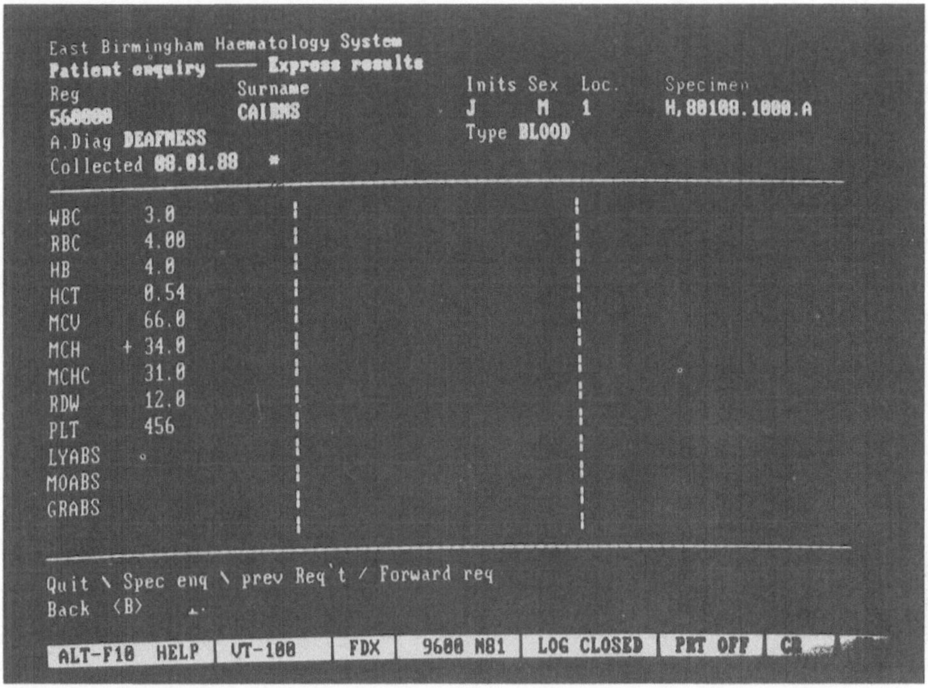

Fig. 13.2. Patient's laboratory data.

morphology and maturation. The common responses are given, each associated with a numeral. An appropriate selection is made, or free text may be entered. The program responds by displaying the chosen answer or free text next to the question for the purpose of verification. In order to speed the process, the default <Enter> or the number "1" key have been made to correspond to the description of the physiological or normal marrow cells. Therefore, if the sample shows little or no abnormality the user can step rapidly through the program using only one or two keys (Fig. 13.3). The response given determines the next screen of questions to be displayed. This branching structure prevents redundant information being sought. For example, if no cells of a given type have been counted, there is little point in asking about their morphology or relation to other cells. The responses are stored and finally used to generate a report. This consists of a template of sentences describing the marrow, with gaps which may be filled by statements governed by the stored responses. The result is a written report which may be stored or printed immediately for checking before issue to the clinicians.

When a detailed differential count of cells is necessary the program designates a defined block of keys so that an individual keystroke is linked to a specific cell type shown on the VDU. These cells are linked together on the screen in two rows relating to the banks of keys: A to H and Z to N. This allows twelve different cell types to be handled and is sufficient for the majority of marrow examinations. The total number necessary for an accurate and reproducible count will vary with the sample and in case of doubt advice is given in the form of help screens. There

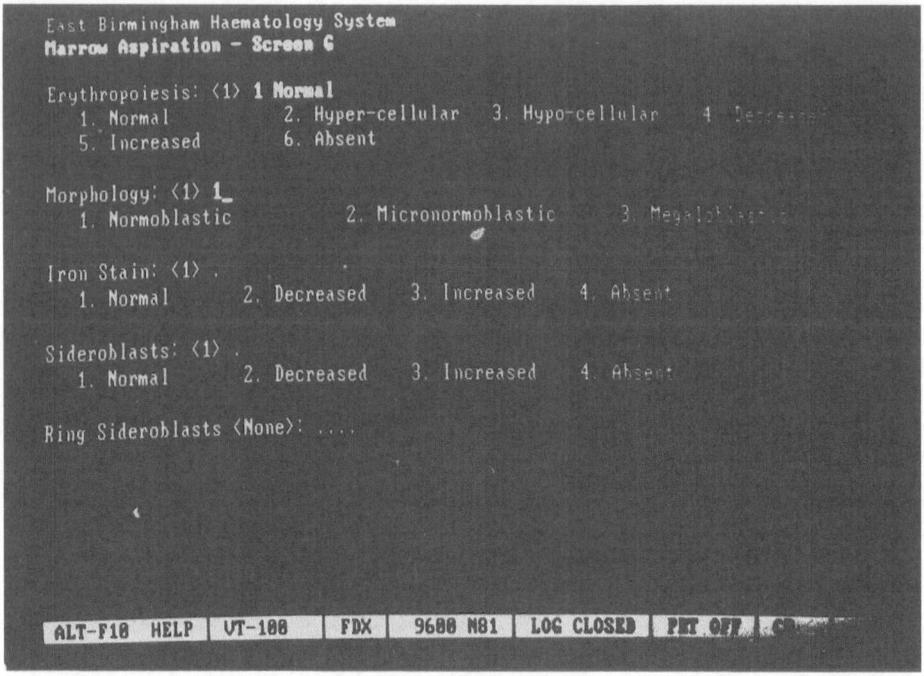

Fig. 13.3. Sample screen from the reporting program.

is no recognised method at present for expressing absolute counts of cells per unit volume of marrow. Considerable variation in numbers of cells may be found in different parts of a slide. When sufficient cells to be representative have been counted, they are recalculated automatically as simple percentages.

Expert System for Assistance in Bone-marrow Reporting

The trainee haematologist is likely to have difficulties in cell recognition and in the early stages will often require help from an experienced microscopist. When this is unavailable computerised guidance can provide assistance in two ways. The first is to return to the menu screen and select the XIP expert system shell (Expertech, 172 Bath Road, Slough, SL1 3XE), which contains an advisory program. Descriptions of cells may be expressed as a set of rules forming the knowledge base of an expert system. These take the general form that if an attribute of a cell has a certain value then a given consequence must follow. In addition, certain facts about number or morphology are expressed as assertions. The program runs by asking a series of questions about the cell that the microscopist cannot recognise. Suggested replies are provided in a similar manner to the parent reporting program. However, these responses are designed to satisfy the conditions (or "if" clauses) of one or more of the knowledge base

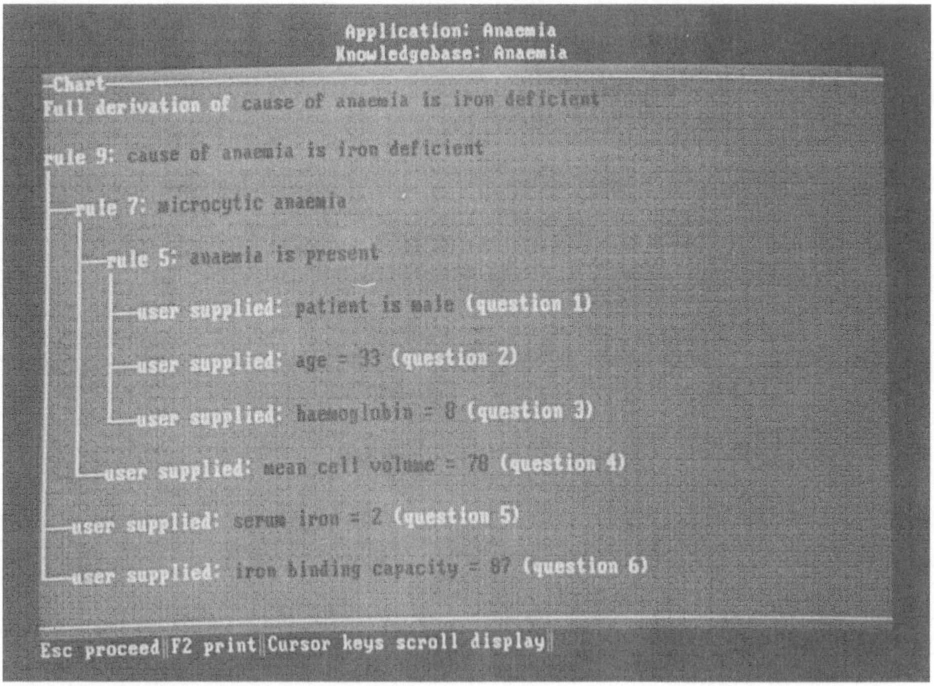

Fig. 13.4. Display of the expert system rules.

rules. The latter having become functional may in turn enable other rules to operate, eventually leading to a conclusion. The sequence of operation is initially to determine whether the cell is undifferentiated. If this is not the case the possibility of belonging to the most frequently occurring differentiated cell line (neutrophilic myeloid) is examined. In the event of failure the next commonest is considered and the process repeated until either the conditions for a postulated line have been satisfied or there are none left for consideration. In the majority of cases the number of possible different cells is relatively small, which should make precise labelling possible. When the cells are malignant and can appear unusually atypical the conclusion is that there is a need for further investigations, which may include identification of cellular antigens, cytochemistry and chromosomes. This program incorporates a charting feature which displays the connected rules and assertions that were used in reaching a conclusion, in hierarchical sequence (Fig. 13.4). Another useful feature is the ability to change items of data and to determine the effect on the conclusions.

Part of the importance of live tuition is the simultaneous viewing of the same optical image, preferably using a double headed microscope. Printed atlases of haematology, though containing a wealth of material, lack the resolution of the originals. Transparencies may be of better quality but are less convenient to view. Microfiches are easier to handle but often of marginal quality. We have transferred examples of normal morphology and abnormal variations from our library of photographic slides through the necessary intermediary stage of videotape onto videodisc. Each frame on the disc has an associated index number

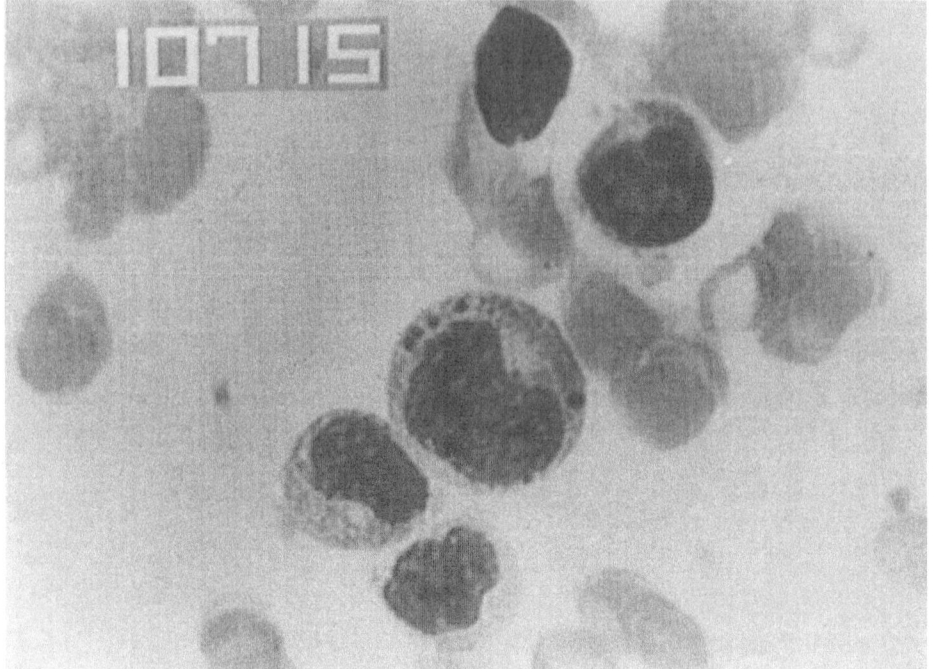

Fig. 13.5. Index cell from slide library.

and may be called up manually by this means. The microscopist uses the expert system to enter findings and to receive the available conclusions including the appropriate index number enabling the example to be shown. This may confirm the initial identification or may call for further thought. As an alternative, the expert system provides the facility for accessing a compatible player directly. It is possible to access the videodisc system directly to use it as a haematological atlas. A menu of all the available cells can be consulted on screen and used to call up the required examples by their index number (Fig. 13.5).

Image Processing Capabilities

The microscope reporting described is subjective and semi-quantitative in nature. An attempt to overcome these restrictions has been made by incorporating image processing and analysis. The MicroScale IIR (Digithurst, 7 Church Lane, Royston, Herts., SG8 9LG) system provides a framestore which accepts the image from a monochrome television camera attached to a second microscope and is connected to a microcomputer. The image from the cameras may be switched from the monitor to a U-matic videorecorder. This allows recording of colour images for later demonstration or possible transfer to a videodisc. The monochrome computer processed images may be stored on videotape, saving

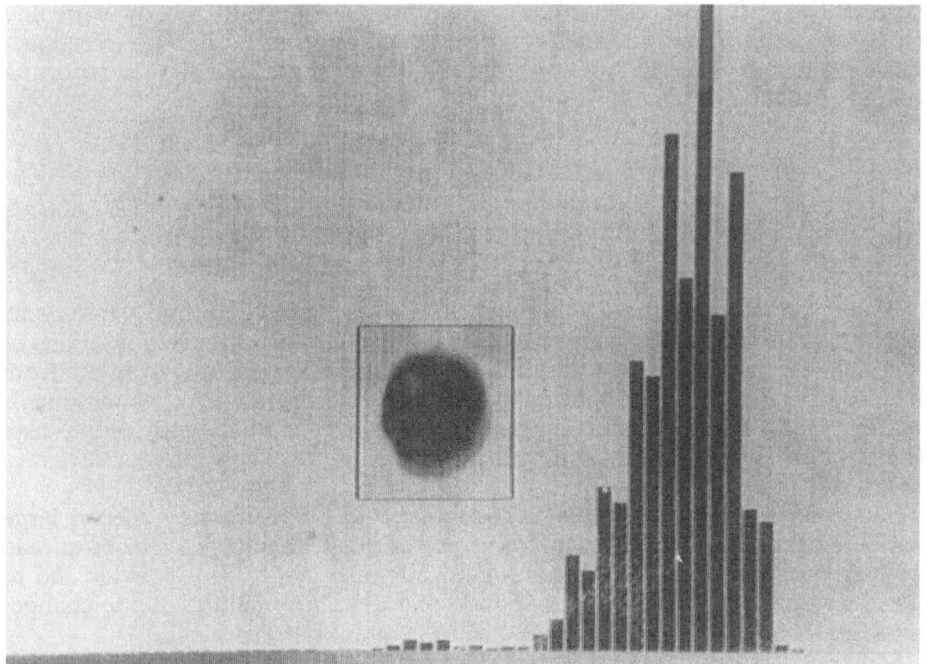

Fig. 13.6. Enhanced image of marrow cell.

computer disc storage capacity. The various functions are displayed on a menu, which is accessed by the mouse. The first task is to capture a frame by pressing the mouse button when a suitable microscope field is in focus. It is possible to count as well as to measure lengths, diameters, perimeters and to calculate areas of objects. By focusing on a graticule of known dimensions the microscope lenses may be calibrated and arbitrary measurements converted into standard units. The intensity may be measured at a point or over an area of the image and may yield alternative information about cellularity. A hard copy of the image may be produced by a standard dot-matrix printer, using the principle of error diffusion with some loss of contrast. We are now in a position to replace subjective statements concerning cell size, shape, intensity and number with precise measurements (Fig. 13.6). The print-out of the results or the image may be useful for follow-up when early changes in cell morphology are being sought. Absolute cell counts per unit area of a marrow biopsy may be calculated instead of being left as percentages.

Experience of the Reporting System

The program, used primarily as a teaching routine, has saved secretarial time and reduced transcription errors by eliminating hand-written and dictated reports.

Experienced staff have criticised the system for its inflexibility, partly overcome by the free text option. The shell can be adapted to provide different questions, answers and templates to suit any user. This also means that similar reporting facilities could be obtained with this program in other disciplines.

Future Development

The next step is to build a database where the rules are conditional statements describing the known consequences of qualitative and quantitative variations of the cell lines. The responses will satisfy some of the rules resulting in advice from the program that may be viewed before the interpretation or conclusion is written. Good quality colour images can be stored in single copy video discs which, when used in conjunction with a microcomputer, allow interactive text to be inserted.

Image processing and simple analyses need to be verified by use on large numbers of cases. A novel macroscopic use of this technology has been to read erythrocyte sedimentation rates automatically at regular time intervals and to plot the resultant slopes. This technique separates abnormalities due to changes in haematocrit from those associated with inflammatory disease.

Some modification to the system is required to allow quicker changes between programs. The main problem is the need to shut down each activity and return to the menu before calling up the next task. A possible solution is further to upgrade to the 80386 series of microprocessors and to run the Microsoft Windows 386 or equivalent program, which should allow multi-tasking. An increase in resident memory will hold all these programs and allow the user to move freely between them.

Alternative methods of data entry include touch-sensitive pads, screens or selection using a mouse may speed data entry.

Acknowledgement. The purchase of the computer and image analysis equipment was made possible by a grant from the Leukaemia Research Fund, UK. The reporting program shell was written in DSM11 MUMPS by members of the Computer Section of the Wolfson Research Laboratories, University of Birmingham, Edgbaston.

References

Clark I, Gyde OHB, Holtom DB (1985) Microcomputer program for cell counting. J Clin Pathol 38: 954–959

14 A Standard Microcomputer System for Patient-Controlled Analgesia Research

Hilary A. Aitken, G.N.C. Kenny and C.S. McArdle

Introduction

There is increasing interest in the use of computerised systems for the control of physiological variables. Where there is a measurable target or end point for the variable such as blood pressure or temperature, then it should be possible to program a computer to maintain the variable close to a predetermined target value. Pain is a subjective and varying phenomenon, and specification of the end point in a form which the computer can recognise is not possible. Patient-controlled analgesia (PCA) is a technique which allows individual patients to titrate suitable doses of analgesic in response to their own assessment of the degree of pain experienced. There are two main advantages of PCA. Firstly, it provides good quality analgesia which is tailored to individual patient requirements. Secondly, because of this, examination of analgesic consumption can provide a reasonable estimate of the amount of pain experienced by patients. Thus it is a useful research tool.

History of Patient-Controlled Analgesia

Most patients who have undergone surgery will require parenteral opioids to provide pain relief. The traditional mode of administration is by intramuscular bolus injection with doses given as required, usually with a specified minimum time interval between doses. Anyone who has ever experienced this type of analgesia will know that it can be less than satisfactory. The reason for this is that the active drug levels are not constant. They rise to a peak level soon after administration and then fall slowly. If the doses are given too far apart, the level will fall below the pain threshold before the next dose is given. However, if the second dose is given too soon, a cumulative effect may occur, causing levels to become high enough for dangerous respiratory side effects. Since most doctors and nurses would wish to err on the side of safety, the result is unsatisfactory analgesia for something like one-third to one-half of all postoperative patients (Cronin et al. 1973). This fluctuation in drug levels may be avoided by use of continuous intravenous infusion of opioids. While this may provide better analgesia, it fails to take account of the fact that pain varies from hour to hour in individual patients, and that each patient has a different pain threshold (Tamsen et al. 1979). Cases of respiratory depression have been described with continuous intravenous infusion of opioids (Catling et al. 1980), which suggest that cumulation may occur. Both these modes of analgesic delivery therefore suffer from the rigidity of the regime. Hence the rationale of putting patients in control of their own analgesia was formulated.

Figure 14.1 is a simple representation of the feedback loop involved in PCA. The patient experiences pain and presses the button. This delivers a predetermined dose of analgesic which should, of course, decrease the pain. From early studies it became apparent that patients do not overdose themselves with opioids (Tamsen et al. 1979). They tend to find a balance between an acceptable degree of pain and side effects such as drowsiness or nausea. They are happy to do this in the knowledge that should the pain worsen, they have the means to alleviate it rapidly. Some of the early systems were very simple. Scott (1970) described a system which he had developed in 1964 for use in obstetric analgesia. This consisted of an infusion of pethidine controlled by a spring-loaded clamp which was normally closed. The woman in labour was instructed, when she felt pain, to squeeze the clamp which allowed the drip to run, and to release it when the pain was eased. A safety feature of this system was that if she became drowsy she would relax her grip and the clamp would close, preventing delivery of the analgesic.

The equipment has gradually become more sophisticated and a number of commercial systems are now available which are compact, efficient, and safe. The incorporation of alarm functions and a "lockout period" is standard in most systems. The lockout period is a preselected time interval following administration of a bolus dose during which a second dose cannot be given. This is designed to prevent a second dose being given before the effects of the first have

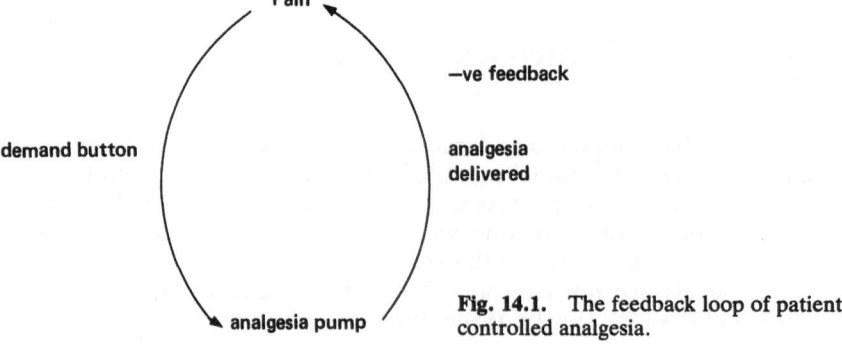

Fig. 14.1. The feedback loop of patient controlled analgesia.

commenced. Some systems also enable a continuous background infusion to be selected in addition to demand bolus doses. Many analgesic drugs have been tried, mostly with success (Harmer et al. 1983; Kay 1981). The only major side effect occurred with buprenorphine where cases of respiratory depression have been described (Gibbs et al. 1982). Although different drugs may have greatly varying durations of action, patients tend to vary the time between doses to compensate for this (Kay 1981). Several routes have been tried, including intravenous, intramuscular (Harmer et al. 1983), and epidural (Sjostrom et al. 1985).

The Glasgow System

PCA can be used as a research tool. Some years ago, workers in the University Department of Anaesthesia at Glasgow Royal Infirmary became interested in the use of PCA in the evaluation of new analgesic drugs. It was realised that groups of patients receiving different analgesic agents could be compared if all groups were, in addition, allowed access to morphine via a PCA system. The amount of morphine requested would provide an objective assessment of the degree of analgesia provided by the trial drugs. It would become ethical to test an analgesic against a placebo, as the patient would still receive satisfactory analgesia from the PCA morphine.

It was found that no existing system was able to store data of the type required; i.e. the number and timing of patient requests. Since data were to be collected for 24 hours, the means of data storage would have to be compact. It was decided to develop a tailor-made system which would meet these requirements. The system is based on an Apple IIe microcomputer linked to an IMED 929 infusion pump (Fig. 14.2). Data are stored on floppy discs and there is also a thermal printer giving hard copy. Since the system is designed for use on general wards and is often moved about, there is a battery back-up.

All the components fit on one trolley and it causes little interference with nursing access to patients, although it is less compact than some of the commercial models. The computer screen continuously displays information about the patient currently using the system, including the bolus dose selected and the total volume infused. There is a selectable lockout period and in addition there are upper dose limits for 1- and 3-hour periods. When the patient's weight is entered, the program calculates a suitable bolus dose, which reduces the risk of prescriber error. Alteration of bolus dose and dose limits is possible only after keyboard entry of a password to prevent unauthorised changes. The microcomputer and infusion pump must communicate with each other at least every 22 seconds. If either component fails to respond within this time, analgesia delivery ceases and an alarm is sounded.

The drug used is morphine, 100 mg in 1000 ml of 0.9% saline, which allows small doses to be given with accuracy. This makes it necessary for an air filter to be incorporated in the analgesia line as small air bubbles form in the delivery tubing, causing the pump alarm to operate. The pump also detects line blockage, and displays appropriate warning and advisory information on the screen as well as sounding an alarm. The analgesia line is connected to the intravenous infusion

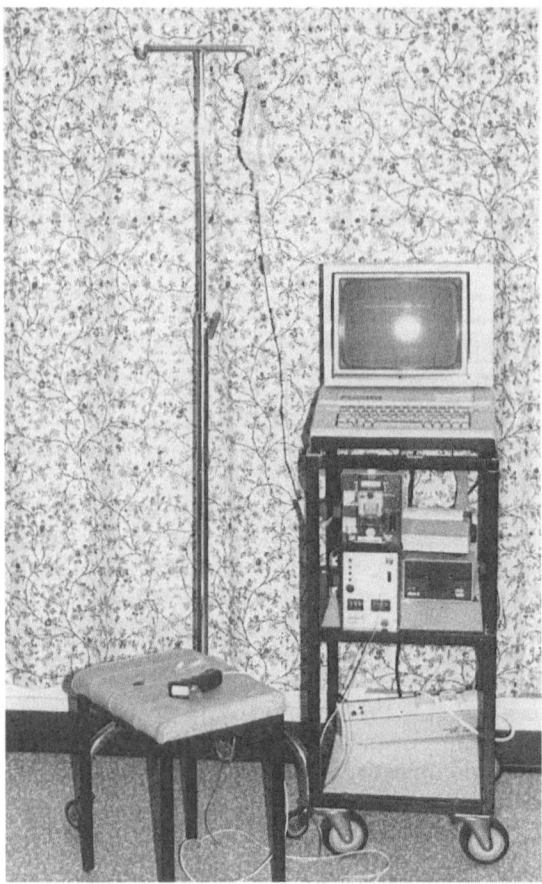

Fig. 14.2.   The Glasgow PCA system.

line. There is a one-way valve (Rosen and Williams 1979) to prevent opioid passing back up the infusion line to form a potentially dangerous reservoir.

The other component of the system is the hand-held button. It was initially designed to respond to a single press, but some of the early patients complained that at times they had pressed the button by accident. It was modified to respond only to two presses within 1 second. Normally a series of bleeps or buzzes informs the patient whether his request has been successful or not, but a speech synthesiser has been incorporated in which a series of statements replace the bleeps (Hodsman et al. 1987b). Most patients preferred this, although some complained about the voice's American accent! So far over 300 patients have used this PCA system with no major complications.

The major concern in design of a PCA system is safety. Most of the safety features of our system have already been mentioned but in summary they are:

Hardware

1. Made from standard components, thus easily maintained and serviced.

2. There are two microprocessors in the system: one in the pump and one in the computer which continuously check on each other
3. Reliable over long periods of operation in contrast with other systems (Owen et al. 1986)
4. Double button push required
5. One-way valve in infusion line

Software
1. Normally only patient weight and age need be entered in set-up program; simplicity reduces operator error
2. Drug bolus doses and dose limits calculated from patient weight
3. Password required to make any changes once system is in operation

The program is versatile; it has been used principally to deliver on-demand bolus doses alone, but it can deliver, in addition, a background infusion. This may run either at a preselected constant rate or at a variable rate which is automatically adjusted every 15 minutes according to the number of bolus demands over the preceding hour. The program can also operate a second pump, which allows the trial drug or placebo to be given automatically. This has been used to give intermittent intramuscular bolus doses of trial drug or placebo.

Other monitors can be linked to the basic system. So far an automatic blood-pressure monitor and an inductance-type respiratory rate monitor have been added for the purposes of specific studies which required data of this type. The data are stored on the same disc as the analgesia data, which enables large amounts of information to be stored in a compact fashion. The same equipment can be used to undertake analysis of analgesia data with a separate analysis program, and can produce graphs of morphine consumption such as the ones illustrated later in Figs. 14.3 to 14.6.

The ordinary Apple IIe microcomputer in this system can revert to other use when not being employed for analgesia studies.

Results

A number of studies have been completed using the equipment and several more are in progress. The system has been found to be reliable and safe, and accurately to record and reproduce data. It is popular with patients, who appreciate being given control of their own analgesia, and with nursing staff, who are relieved of the time-consuming task of checking and administering opioid analgesics. The patients, on the whole, rapidly understand and become confident with the system. Elderly patients occasionally have difficulty using it satisfactorily, and it has been found that very anxious patients may use it incorrectly in an attempt to relieve fear rather than pain.

The morphine consumption pattern of patients using PCA morphine alone confirmed the findings of previous investigators in that there was an enormous variation in the amount used. Figure 14.3 shows a plot of cumulative morphine

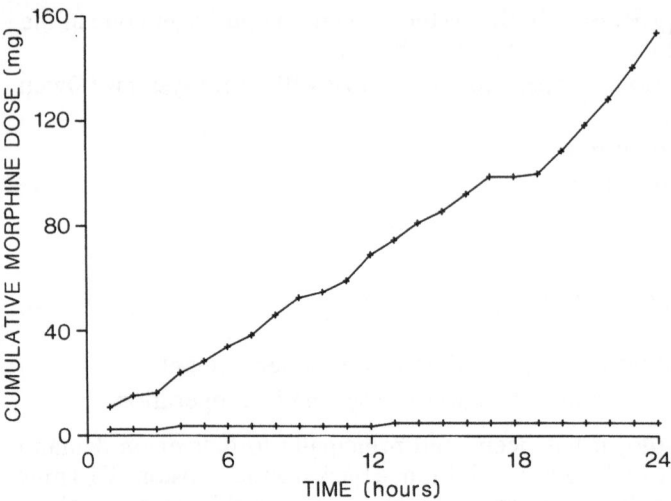

Fig. 14.3. Cumulative morphine consumption of two patients. Total 24-hour doses are 154 mg and 5.2 mg.

consumption over 24 hours for two patients and illustrates this finding. One patient required 30 times more morphine than the other despite the fact that both patients were male, of similar age and weight, and both had had upper abdominal surgery.

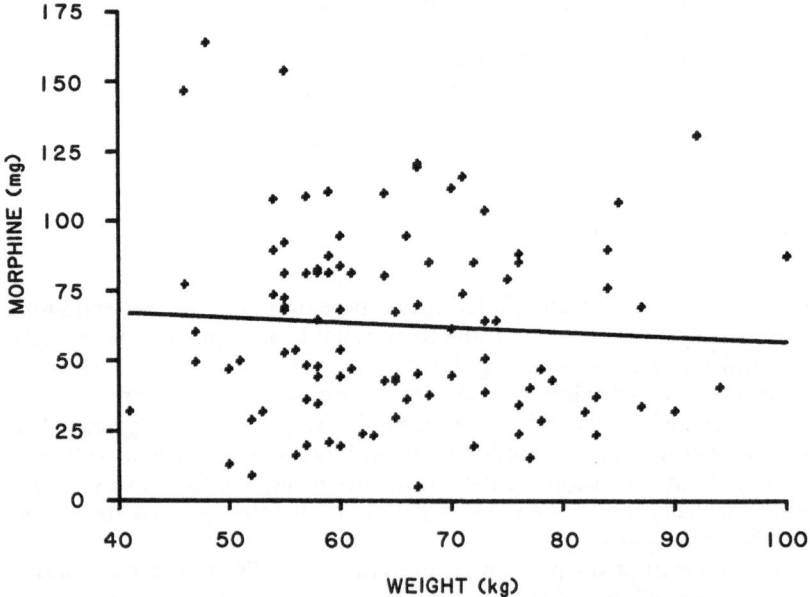

Fig. 14.4. Total 24-hour morphine requirement plotted against weight for 100 patients.

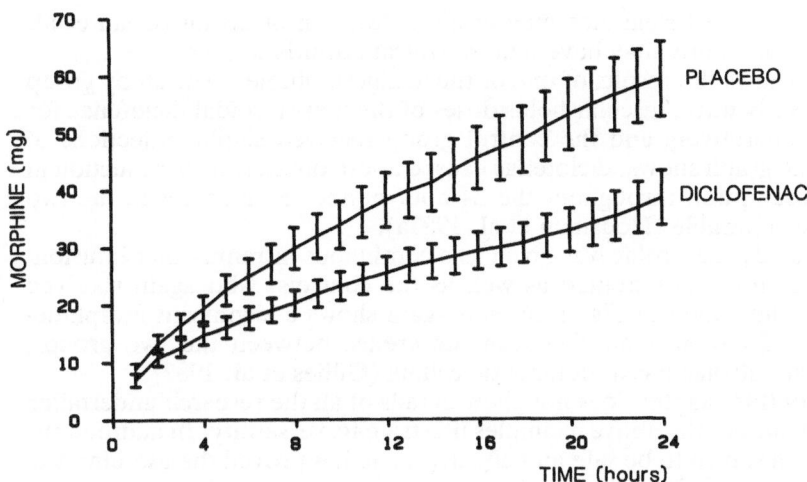

Fig. 14.5. Cumulative morphine consumption; diclofenac versus placebo. (Hodsman et al. 1987a: reproduced by kind permission of the authors and the editor of *Anaesthesia*).

The variation is seen again in Fig. 14.4, in which the total morphine consumption over 24 hours is plotted against weight for 100 patients. No correlation was found, which indicates the irrationality of current prescribing practices (Burns et al. 1988).

When morphine consumption was plotted against age, a negative correlation was found. There are a number of reasons why this may be the case. It has been suggested that reduced opioid binding may give an apparent increase in plasma

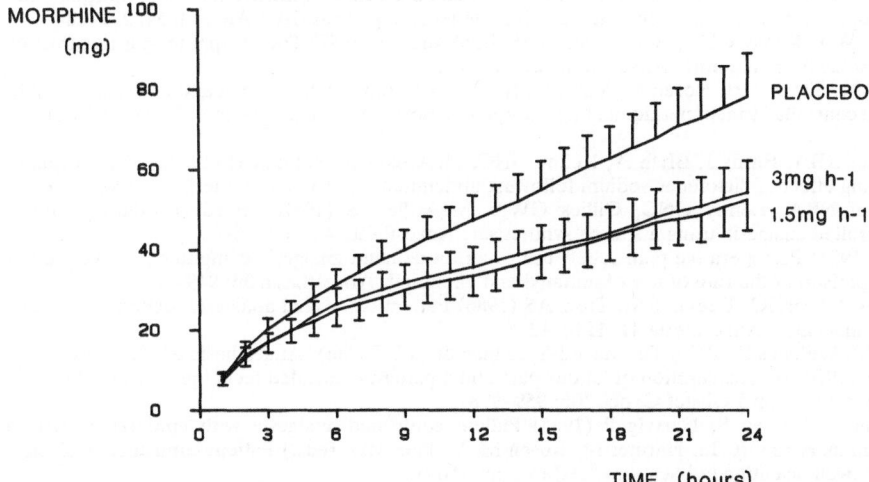

Fig. 14.6. Cumulative morphine consumption; ketorolac (two infusion rates) versus placebo. (Gillies et al. 1987: reproduced by kind permission of the authors and the editor of *Anaesthesia*).

concentration, reduced clearance may prolong duration of action (Chan et al. 1975), or that the elderly may have a more stoical attitude to pain.

Figure 14.5 shows the results of one of the analgesic studies. The study group received 12-hourly intramuscular bolus doses of the non-steroidal diclofenac for 24 hours postoperatively and the control group received similar injections of placebo. As the graph shows, diclofenac caused approximately 30% reduction in morphine consumption throughout the 24-hour period. Pain scores in the two groups were comparable (Hodsman et al. 1987a).

In another study, ketorolac was given as a continuous intramuscular infusion. Two dosage groups were studied as well as the controls, who again received saline. This is illustrated in Fig. 14.6, and again shows a significant morphine-sparing effect. There was no significant difference between the two groups, suggesting that ketrolac has a therapeutic ceiling (Gillies et al. 1987).

The scope of this chapter does not allow details of all the research undertaken using this system, but the above examples illustrate its versatility. In addition the system has been shown to be safe and effective, and has proved the usefulness of PCA as a way of assessing other analgesic agents.

References and Further Reading

Bahar M, Rosen M, Vickers MD (1985) Self-administered nalbuphine, morphine, and pethidine: comparison by intravenous route following cholecystectomy. Anaesthesia 40: 529–532

Burns JW, Hodsman NBA, McLintock TA, Gillies GWA, Kenny GNC, McArdle CS (1988) The influence of patient characteristics on the requirements for postoperative analgesia. Anaesthesia (in press)

Chan K, Kendal MJ, Mitchard M, Wells WDE, Vickers MD (1975) The effect of ageing on plasma pethidine concentration. Br J Clin Pharmac 2: 297–302

Cronin M, Redfern PA, Utting JE (1973) Psychometry and postoperative complaints in surgical patients. Br J Anaesth 45: 879–886

Catling JA, Pinto DM, Jordan C, Jones JG (1980) Respiratory effects of analgesia after cholecystectomy: comparison of continuous and intermittent papaveretum. Br Med J 281: 478–484

Gibbs JM, Johnson HD, Davis FM (1982) Patient administration of intravenous buprenorphine for postoperative pain relief using the "Cardiff" demand apparatus. Br J Anaesth 54: 279–284

Gillies GWA, Kenny GNC, Bullingham RES, McArdle CS (1987) The morphine sparing effect of ketorolac tromethamine. Anaesthesia 42: 727–731

Harmer M, Slattery PJ, Rosen M, Vickers MD (1983) Intramuscular on demand analgesia: double blind controlled trial of pethidine, buprenorphine, morphine, and meptazinol. Br Med J 286: 680–682

Hodsman NBA, Burns J, Blyth A, Kenny GNC, McArdle CS, Rotman H (1987a) The morphine sparing effect of diclofenac sodium following abdominal surgery. Anaesthesia 42: 1005–1008

Hodsman NBA, Kenny GNC, Gillies GWA, McArdle CS (1987b) Feedback during patient controlled analgesia using a speech synthesiser. Anaesthesia 42: 767–769

Kay B (1981) Postoperative pain relief: use of an on demand analgesic computer (ODAC) and a comparison of the rate of use of fentanyl and alfentanil. Anaesthesia 36: 949–951

Owen H, Glavin RJ, Reekie RM, Trew AS (1986) Patient controlled analgesia: experience of two new machines. Anaesthesia 41: 1230–1235

Rosen M, Williams B (1979) The valved-Y-connector (VYC Con). Anaesthesia 34: 882–884

Scott JS (1970) A consideration of labour pain and a patient-controlled technique for its relief with meperidine. Am J Obstet Gynec 106: 959–978

Sjostrom S, Tamsen S, Hartvig P (1985) Patient controlled analgesia with epidural opiates: a preliminary report. In: Harmer M, Rosen M, Vickers MD, (eds.) Patient controlled analgesia. Blackwell Scientific Publications, Oxford, pp. 156–159

Tamsen A, Hartvig P, Dahlstrom B, Lindstrom B, Holmdahl MH (1979) Patient controlled analgesia in the early postoperative period. Acta Anaesth Scand 23: 462–470

15 Control of Unstable Blood Pressure using a Modified Negative Feedback System

B.E. Keogh

Introduction

The development of the heart–lung machine combined with the ability to induce reversible asystole during surgery has allowed cardiac surgery to evolve into a major specialty over the last 30 years. Improvements in myocardial preservation, anaesthetic techniques and immediate postoperative management have resulted in a significant reduction in perioperative mortality. Hypertension is a common postoperative problem, particularly following coronary artery bypass grafting when it may occur in up to 70% of patients. The prime cause for the hypertension is increased peripheral vascular resistance due in part to the pathophysiological effects of cardiopulmonary bypass and in part due to the hypothermia which is induced during cardiopulmonary bypass to optimise organ preservation. Hypertension is undesirable because it threatens fresh anastamoses and increases myocardial work (Estafanous and Tarazi 1980). It is characterised by occurrence in the first few postoperative hours, a paroxysmal course, a mild tachycardia and an elevated mean rate of left ventricular ejection with an associated increase in myocardial oxygen consumption.

A logical approach towards antihypertensive therapy in this setting is the administration of potent vasodilators to reduce the peripheral vascular resistance and hence the blood pressure. In recent years sodium nitroprusside infusion (SNP) has gained wide acceptance as the vasodilator of choice. The standard method of administration of SNP is via a volumetric infusion pump which is controlled manually by the attending intensive care unit (ICU) nurse. In unstable patients a considerable proportion of the nurse's time is demanded in making moment-to-moment adjustments of the infusion rate to avoid catastrophic fluctuations in arterial pressure. The nurse-time required is sometimes at the expense of other vital activities and this has stimulated interest in closing the control loop with a computer. However, the development of software to drive such a system reliably has been complicated by the fact that sodium nitroprusside has a delayed onset of action of 20–30 seconds and a half life of 1–2 minutes. This

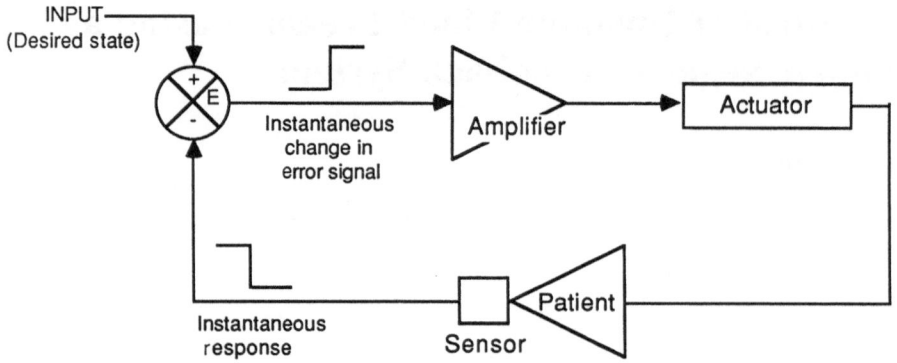

a *Without lag in system*

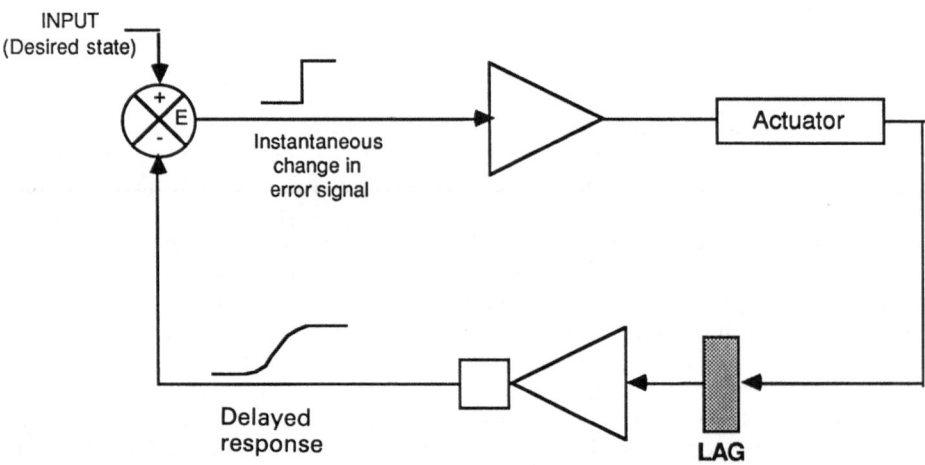

b *With lag in system*

Fig. 15.1. With ideal negative feedback loop a change in the existing state of the system is corrected immediately (*a*). If a lag is introduced, e.g. delayed onset of action of sodium nitroprusside, then the correction is delayed (*b*).

is further complicated by 10-fold variation in patient sensitivity, not only between patients but also in the same patient at different times (Slate, 1980). In addition, any reliable software should effectively filter arterial waveform artefacts. Following the pioneering work of Sheppard (1980) a variety of custom-made closed-loop systems have been applied to this problem (Potter et al. 1984; de Asla et al. 1985; Rosenfeldt et al. 1986; Reid and Kenny 1987). These systems were based on a simple negative feedback loop between arterial pressure and infusion rate of the

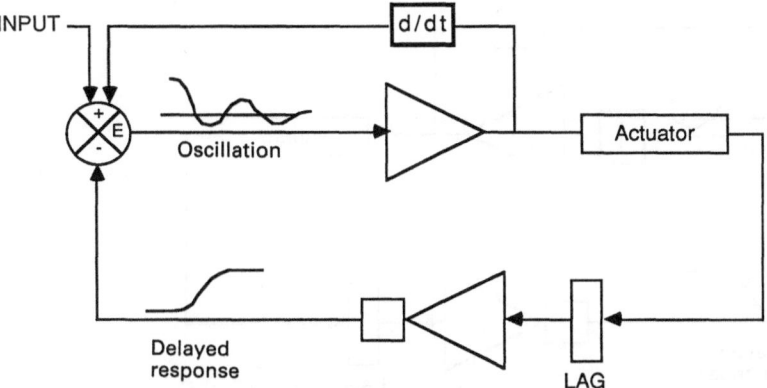

Fig. 15.2. A delayed response in a simple loop will result in over-correction of the error with oscillation until a steady state is reached. This can be reduced by introducing a derivative circuit which reduces the signal to the actuator as the error returns to zero, thus reducing the tendency to over-correction.

vasodilator and hence are theoretically subject to the problem of oscillation resulting primarily from the delayed onset of action of SNP in a constantly changing environment.

The principles of a simple negative feedback loop are shown in Fig. 15.1. A transducer senses the existing state of a system (in this case the blood pressure) and converts it to an electronic signal which is passed to a central processing unit where it is compared with the desired state of the system (desired blood pressure). The difference between the two is known as the error. The error signal is amplified so as to drive an actuator (in this case an infusion pump) which will alter the system in such a way as to reduce the error to zero. When the error is instantaneous and the response instantaneous, such a system is very effective. However, in the case of blood pressure control the delayed onset of action of SNP results in a 20–30-second lag in the system which, combined with the prolonged duration of action of SNP (half-life of 2 minutes), can result in over-correction and oscillation in a rapidly changing physiological environment. This tendency can be reduced by introducing a derivative feedback loop into the control circuit (Fig. 15.2). The derivative loop analyses the amplified error signal which is driving the actuator and influences the signal in such a way as to reduce the rate of return to zero as the error becomes less, thereby reducing the chance of an over-correction. Such a circuit is known as a proportional plus derivative feedback loop. Although oscillation is the main source of error all feedback loops will have some small degree of error which will become more apparent with time. Such "creepage" can be reduced by the introduction of an integral circuit to form a proportional plus integral plus derivative (PID) feedback loop (Fig. 15.3).

Such principles have been employed in industry since the 1950s; the commonest example of the application of a PID loop is the computer disc drive. If the head is reading information from disc track 79 and needs to retrieve further data from track 9 then it sweeps across the disc towards track 9, initially at maximum speed, but as it approaches track 9 the sweep slows under the influence of a derivative circuit, until it stops over track 9.

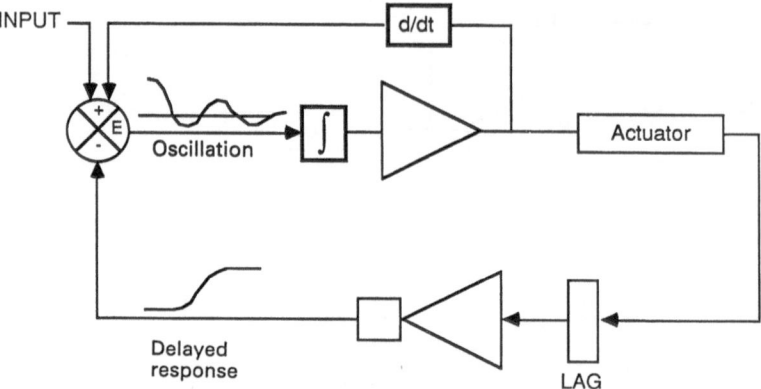

Fig. 15.3. The introduction of an integral circuit enables correction of the tendency towards error within the circuit itself.

The application of such technology to medicine has had to await the advent of microprocessors which can easily be accommodated in manageable-sized bedside modules.

We assessed the research prototype of a closed loop regulator (IVAC Titrator Model 10K) based on a PID feedback loop to improve the quality of postoperative mean arterial pressure (MAP) control. The unit was a self-contained module, not much larger than a standard IVAC volumetric pump, which could be mounted on a drip stand. It was designed to interface with the IVAC 560 volumetric pump in current usage. The analogue arterial signal from a transducer connected to an indwelling arterial cannula was passed to the IVAC Titrator which looked at the signal without interruption and passed it unaltered to the usual remote monitor.

The analogue signal as seen by the Titrator was then passed to an analogue to digital converter (ADC). The digital output from the ADC was analysed over every 10-second period to derive, by integration, the actual MAP. On the basis of this MAP, together with the desired MAP (entered by the attending nurse or physician) and infusion rate over the same period, a new infusion rate for the following 10 seconds was calculated. Thus the central algorithm was executed every 10 seconds.

Automatic infusion of the SNP was initiated with a transient controller module. This module was designed to keep the patient's MAP on a smooth trajectory to the desired level. During this initial period the infusion rate was calculated according to the MAP error (the difference between the actual and desired MAP) and velocity of error (also referred to as phase plane analysis).

Once the patient's MAP was controlled near the desired MAP (30 sec to 8 min 20 sec) a linear controller was invoked to maintain steady, oscillation-free control. In this module the calculation of the infusion rate was based on the classical feedback control concept of a proportional plus integral plus derivative negative feedback loop. The algorithm was continuously modified by a series of peripheral software modules designed to respond to patient variables. The two most important of these modules were the artefact detector, designed to identify non-physiological pressure waveforms, and the patient gain compensation multiplier, which influenced the infusion rate according to the patient's dose–response curve based on the immediately preceding 24-minute record.

Two cohorts of cardiac surgery patients requiring SNP for postoperative hypertension (MAP >70 mm Hg) were studied prospectively. In the first cohort of 12 patients hypertension was controlled by manual adjustment of the infusion rate of a Vickers volumetric pump by the attending ICU nurse. Blood pressure was monitored by a Gould P50 transducer via a radial arterial line. The analogue signal from the transducer was passed to a remote monitor where the signal was converted to a digital display of mean arterial pressure. The nurse was asked to maintain a MAP of 70 mm Hg. The analogue signal was also passed to the IVAC Titrator where an analogue to digital converter (ADC) obtained 100 samples per second enabling accurate calculation of the MAP. The actual MAP over consecutive 10-second periods was passed via a RS232 interface to a floppy disc file for subsequent analysis. During this phase of the study the Titrator was used only for its facility to calculate the MAP and to write this to disc, and to allow the nursing staff to become familiar with the user interface of the Titrator.

In the second cohort of 22 patients blood pressure was controlled automatically using the closed loop Titrator system to adjust the rate of SNP infusion to maintain the desired MAP of 70 mm Hg.

In both groups specific information regarding blood pressure and infusion status for each 10-second period throughout the period of SNP infusion was recorded onto a floppy disc, creating 99 496 data-points in the Titrator group and 56 273 data-points in the manual group.

These data were compared with the desired MAP setpoint as entered by the attending nurse.

Efficacy of Computer Control

The mean arterial pressure in both groups was comparable prior to the commencement of SNP infusion.

Data analysis showed the amount of time the patient's MAP was within a specific range when compared with the desired MAP. The five ranges were Very Low (less than -20% below the setpoint), Low (-20% to -10% below the setpoint), within 10% of the setpoint, High (10% to 20% above the setpoint) and Very High (greater than 20% above the setpoint).

Table 15.1 shows the overall MAP point distribution within the five pressure ranges. Each point represents a 10-second period.

The desired pressure range was considered to be within 10% of the setpoint and the aim in both groups was to keep the patient's MAP within this range. The results show that the IVAC Titrator maintained the MAP within the desired range 90% of the time as compared with 45.8% under manual control. In addition there is a positive skew towards high blood pressure in the manual group, with these patients spending 37.2% of the time at a MAP greater than the desired range, as opposed to the Titrator-controlled group who only spent 6.4% of the time above the desired MAP.

Each patient was analysed for each of 12 mutually exclusive time frames of 10 minutes during the first 2 hours of infusion. The percent error for each 10-second interval for each patient was calculated according to the following formula:

Table 15.1. The mean arterial pressure (MAP) of consecutive 10-second periods during sodium nitroprusside infusion was recorded as a datum point. The distribution of these points in relation to the desired MAP is shown

	Overall point distribution				
	Very low >20%	Low	Within 10%	High	Very high >20%
Titrator group					
Point distribution	718	2801	89545	4593	1839
% distribution	0.7%	2.8%	90.0%	4.6%	1.8%
Manual group					
Point distribution	2950	6586	25775	11225	9736
% distribution	5.2%	2.8%	45.8%	19.9%	17.3%

$$\text{Percent error} = \frac{\text{Actual MAP} - \text{Desired MAP}}{\text{Desired MAP}}$$

The mean percent error for each 10-minute time frame for every patient was established. This created a data-point for each individual patient-time frame. The mean percent errors for each time frame in each group are shown (Fig. 15.4). The results showed that while the IVAC Titrator reduced the mean percent error to about 5% during the second 10 minutes, the nurse-controlled group had still not reached this level after 2 hours.

Repeated measures analysis of variance using the mean percent errors for each patient in each time frame during the first 2 hours of SNP infusion confirmed that there was a significant reduction in error with time in both groups ($p < 0.01$) and that the error in the Titrator group was significantly less than in the manual group ($p < 0.01$).

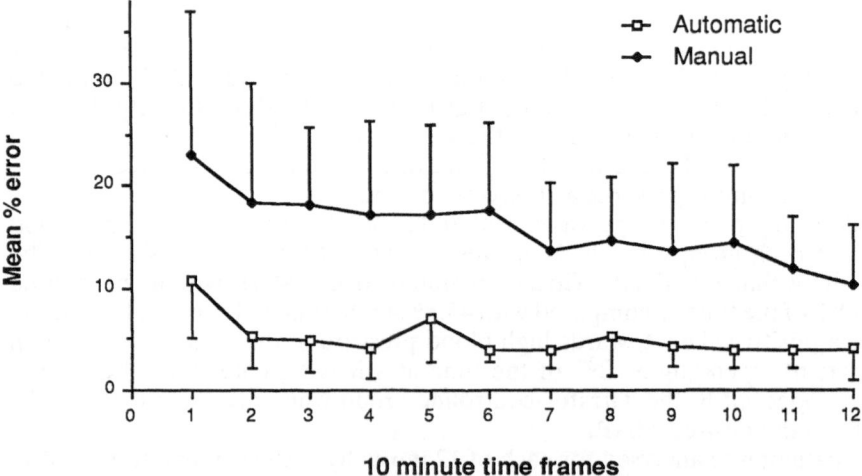

Fig. 15.4. The error of blood pressure control in each group is shown as the mean percent error (±SD) calculated over 10-minute intervals during the first 2 hours of sodium nitroprusside infusion.

Perspectives

This study showed that the closed loop system was more effective than ICU nurses in maintaining mean arterial blood pressure within predefined limits. This was probably due to two main features of the closed loop system. First, the MAP was calculated by integration every 10 seconds and the control algorithm executed accordingly; secondly, the program automatically and continuously modified its response sensitivity every 10 seconds according to the patient's dose–response curve and trends over the preceding 24 minutes.

Several routines contributed to the overall safety of the system. Firstly, the IVAC Titrator verified the functional status of the pump at a minimum frequency of once every 3 seconds; secondly, artefacts were filtered out by comparing the pressure waveform to a range of physiologically possible waveform characteristics thus allowing the Titrator to ignore momentary interruptions of a specific waveform (e.g. flushing arterial line, withdrawal of blood samples). If such an interruption continued for 120 seconds an alarm sounded. In our experience the artefact detector was extremely efficient. Finally, if the MAP dropped to 75% of the desired MAP then the infusion of SNP was immediately discontinued.

A chart from the printer of the Titrator prototype (Fig. 15.5) which shows patient and Titrator responses to a bolus dose of a second potent vasodilator illustrates another important difference between rigid algorithm control and

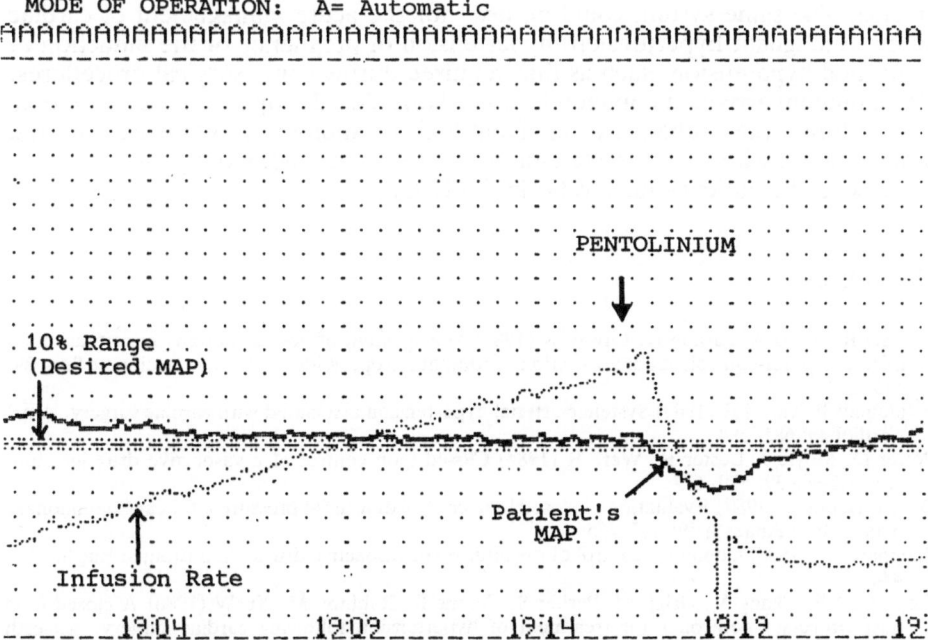

Fig. 15.5. A print-out from the IVAC Titrator showing the effect of a potent vasdilator (pentolinium) on the mean arterial pressure (MAP) and the resultant automatic reduction of sodium nitroprusside infusion rate.

manual control. Following the injection of pentolinium the MAP falls precipitously, and the infusion rate decreases until the infusion is switched off automatically, when the MAP reaches 75% of the desired level. However, the infusion recommences as soon as the MAP rises above the 75% limit, even though the MAP is still below the desired level. This facilitates a smooth return to the desired range without overshoot. Observation of ICU practices confirms that in manually-controlled patients the infusion of SNP is seldom recommenced while the MAP remains depressed, thus increasing the tendency to oscillation and, as a result, MAP overshoot. This may also partly explain the skew to higher pressures in the nurse-controlled group. Other factors contributing towards the increased MAP in the manual group are the length of time taken to control the MAP after commencement of SNP infusion when multiple demands are placed on the attending nurse during the patient's initial "settling in" period, and the tendency of even experienced ICU nurses, particularly when overworked, to feel more reassured with the blood pressure slightly elevated than depressed.

In view of the limited availability of suitably qualified nurses for intensive care posts, verification of the effectiveness and safety of such a system has wide-reaching implications in terms of patient management and deployment of senior and junior nursing staff within the ICU. Relegation of this repetitive and well-defined task to a computer allows greater freedom of nursing at the bedside. When combined with a print-out of blood pressure and infusion rate it reduces time spent on frequent up-dating of charts, and reduces the problem of missing data due to distraction, oversight or excessive workload. Although the concept of closed loop control of hypertension has been developed within the well-documented sphere of postsurgical hypertension its potential application is diverse. The same system could be used for the acute management of cardiac failure, malignant hypertension, hypertension of pregnancy or the induction of controlled hypotension, such as that required during some surgical procedures. The imminent arrival of commercially available closed loop systems should force us to address the problems of applying high technology to mundane but vital nursing tasks, with the ultimate aim of increasing productivity by facilitating an increase in the patient–nurse ratio in the ICU.

References

de Asla R, Benis A, Jurado R, Litwak R (1985) Management of postcardiotomy hypertension by microcomputer-controlled administration of sodium nitroprusside. J Thorac Cardiovasc Surg 89: 115–120

Estafanous F, Tarazi R (1980) Systemic arterial hypertension associated with cardiac surgery. Am J Cardiol 46: 685–694

Potter D, Moyle J, Lester R, Ware R (1984) Closed loop control of a vasoactive drug infusion. Anaesthesia 39: 670–677

Reid J, Kenny G (1987) Evaluation of closed loop control of arterial pressure after cardiopulmonary bypass. Br J Anaesth 59: 247–255

Sheppard LC (1980) Computer control of the infusion of vasoactive drugs. Ann Biomed Eng 8: 431–444

Rosenfeldt F, Chang V, Grigg M, Parker S, Cearns R, Rabinov M, Xu W (1986) A closed loop microprocessor controller for treatment of hypertension following cardiac surgery. Anaesth Intens Care 14: 158–162

16 A Computer-Controlled Hyperthermia System

S.W. Hughes, J.E. Saunders and A.R. Timothy

Introduction

Hyperthermia, raised temperature, has been used as a means of treating cancer for centuries. Hippocrates (400 BC) and Galen (200 BC) used red-hot irons to treat small tumours. Much later, after the Renaissance, there are many reports of spontaneous tumour regression in patients with fevers produced by erysipelas, malaria, smallpox, tuberculosis and influenza. These illnesses produce fevers of about 40 °C which last for several days. Temperatures of at least 40 °C were found to be necessary for tumour regression. Towards the end of the nineteenth century pyrogenic bacteria were injected into patients with cancer. In 1896, Coley used a mixture of erysipelas and *B. prodigeosus* toxins, with some success.

A systematic investigation of hyperthermia has only been carried out since the beginning of this century. Cancer cells may be more sensitive to heat than normal cells (Westermark 1927). Westermark found that 90 minutes at 45 °C killed tumour cells, while normal cells were unaffected. Subsequently, many tumour cells have been found to be no more thermosensitive than normal cells. Work in the 1970s showed that hyperthermia acts as a radiosensitiser, i.e. increases the sensitivity of cells to radiation damage (Arcangeli 1983). One suggestion is that hyperthermia inhibits the repair of sublethal radiation damage in cells. The critical temperature for this effect appears to be around 42–43 °C. Conner (1977) found that if cancer cells were heated at 43 °C and then given a radiation dose of 600 rads the cell kill was 1000 times greater than at 37 °C.

Heat alone is also thought to kill hypoxic cells more than normoxic cells. Hypoxic cells tend to be further away from blood vessels and to heat up more because less heat is conducted away. A tumour showing the two regions is illustrated schematically, in Fig. 16.1.

Radiation and heat affect normal cells as well as cancer cells, but to a lesser degree. The maximum difference in sensitivity to heat between malignant and normal tissues is thought to occur between 42 °C and 43 °C. Usually the threshold

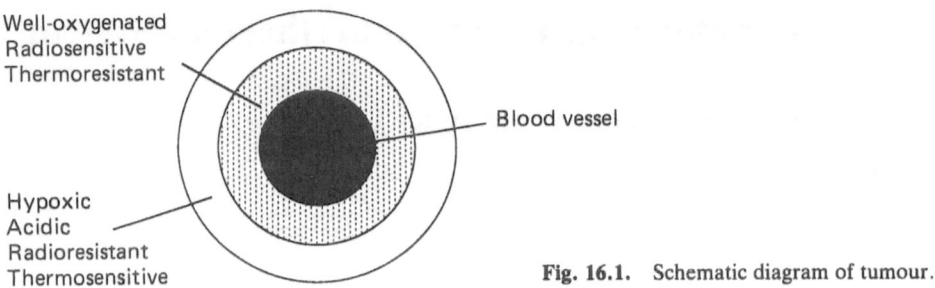

Well-oxygenated
Radiosensitive
Thermoresistant

Blood vessel

Hypoxic
Acidic
Radioresistant
Thermosensitive

Fig. 16.1.   Schematic diagram of tumour.

for hyperthermic damage is taken to be 42.5 °C (Sapareto and Dewey 1984). The purpose of any hyperthermia system is to maintain the tumour temperature at 42.5 °C or above, and the temperature of surrounding normal tissue at below 42.5 °C (Hand and James 1986).

Hardware

The system is shown in Fig. 16.2 and Fig. 16.3. It consists of two principal components; the heating system and the computer system. The heating system

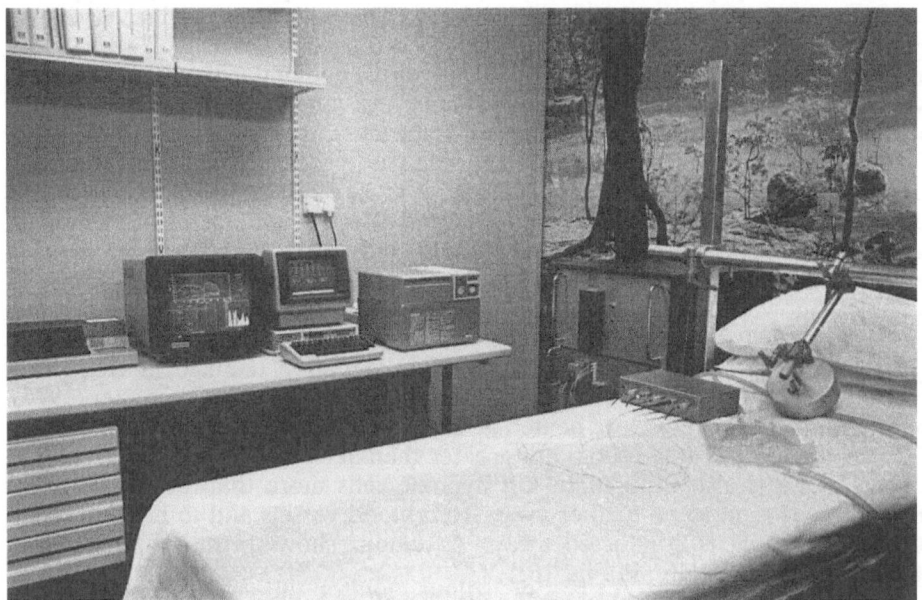

Fig. 16.2.   The treatment room showing the computer system, RF generator system and treatment couch.

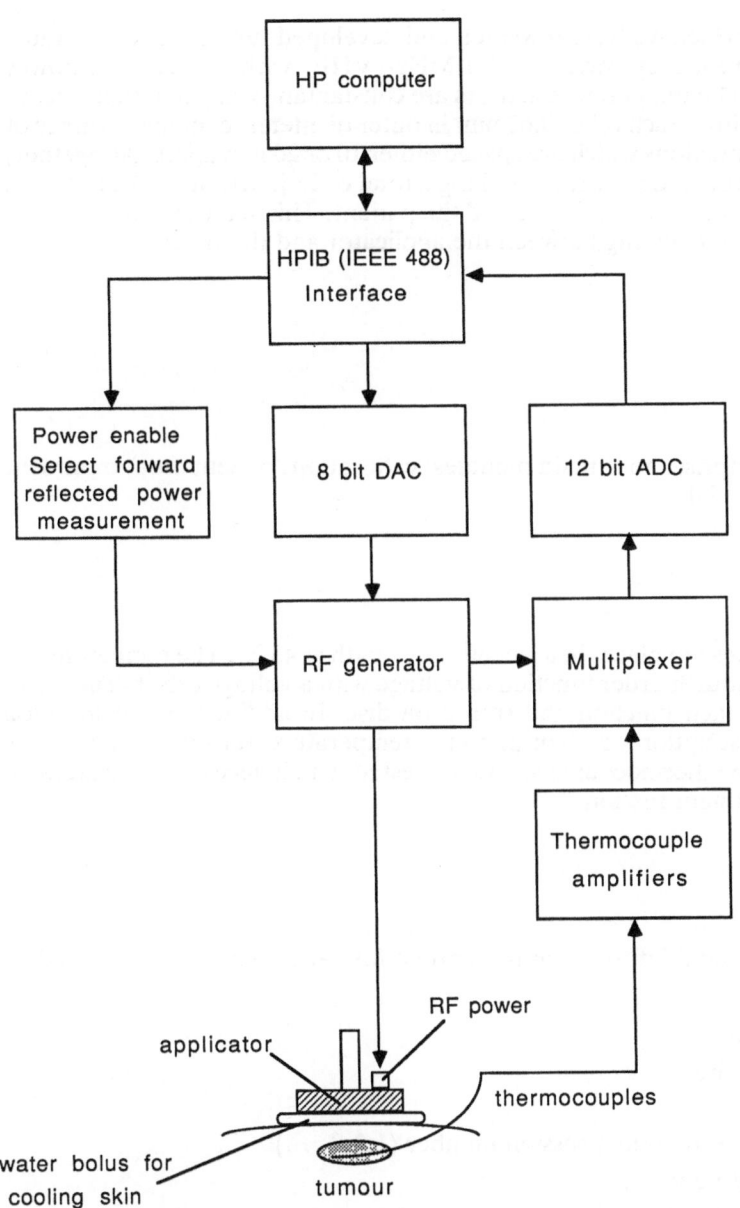

Fig. 16.3. Schematic diagram of the equipment. ADC: analogue to digital converter. DAC: digital-to-analogue converter.

was supplied by Microwave Engineering Design (MED), Newport, Isle of Wight, UK. The computer system is a Hewlett Packard 9816 with two 3.5-inch discs and VDU, an inkjet printer, A3 plotter, colour monitor and an HPIB (IEEE 488) interface. The system was developed by MED in conjunction with the Hammersmith Hospital hyperthermia unit. The system was supplied with a monitoring and control program which we have rewritten and developed further. The generator produces radio frequency waves at 200 MHz (VHF) with a maximum power output of 500W. The temperature sensors are constantan–manganin thermocouples in plastic tubing. Each tube, 0.63 mm in outer diameter, contains an array of 5 thermocouple junctions which are spaced either 10 or 20 mm apart. Altogether, there are five thermocouple arrays, making a total of 25 junctions. A water bolus is interposed between the applicator and the patient. This serves to cool the skin and to improve the coupling between the applicator and the tissue.

Software

The software comprises four main modules: calibration, patient data, treatment and review of the data.

Calibration

The thermocouples are places in a stirred water-bath at 43 °C. The temperature is assumed to be a fourth order function of voltage with a voltage offset. The offset is measured for each junction and stored on disc. In addition, the calibration program has a test option which displays the temperature at each junction every 10 seconds. All the thermocouple arrays are tested, and if necessary, recalibrated before each treatment session.

Patient Data

The following general information is recorded for each treatment and stored on disc:

1. Patient name
2. Hospital number
3. Date of birth
4. Hyperthermia treatment session number (1,2,3. . .)
5. Date of treatment
6. Time of treatment
7. Time interval between radiotherapy and hyperthermia
8. Radiotherapy dose
9. Location of tumour
10. Type of tumour
11. Location of thermocouples (tumour, normal tissue)
12. Name of the data file
13. Disc volume that the file is on

The information module creates a file ready to receive all the treatment data; the patient information is stored in this file. The filename is normally made up from the patient's initials followed by the hyperthermia session number. Information may be entered before or after the treatment is given. A separate program module enables the information to be reviewed and edited at any time.

Treatment

Before treatment commences all of the connected thermocouples are checked by the computer. Any thermocouples that are open circuit are not used to make temperature measurements. The channel numbers of all the working thermocouples, and those not working, are listed on the VDU. The voltage offsets measured by the calibration program are read off the disc and put into an array. These values are added to each corresponding thermocouple measurement to produce the correct temperature reading. During treatment, a temperature–time plot of selected thermocouples is displayed on the colour monitor. This graph may be rescaled during treatment, but initial axis limits are requested before treatment. The default values are 30–50 °C and 0–30 minutes. The treatment program reads the thermocouples, updates the VDU and monitor, adjusts the power, and does various maintenance operations within a predetermined certain cycle time. The cycle time is selected before treatment and is usually 15 seconds. One of the thermocouple junctions is selected as the control thermocouple. The control algorithm tries to maintain this junction at the target temperature. The control thermocouple may be changed at any time during treatment.

A target temperature (normally 43 °C) and the rate of temperature rise at the control thermocouple (normally 1 °C per minute) are set. A faster rate than 1 °C per minute can cause pain, and a slower rate makes the rise time too long. Temperature and power readings are stored on disc every four cycles. The temperature at any five thermocouples may be displayed graphically on the monitor. A whole array may be displayed or a selection made from different arrays. Different junctions may be selected for display at any time during the treatment.

As well as the temperature–time plot on the colour monitor, each temperature is displayed in histogram form (Fig. 16.4). Thermocouple arrays in the tumour are displayed in red (filled columns) and those in normal tissue and on the skin are displayed in yellow (open columns). The array type is specified before treatment. After running through the start-up procedure, a few cycles are allowed to pass to check the temperature readings before the power is switched on. The thermocouples in the tumour or surrounding tissue will be at about 37 °C and those on the skin about 31–36 °C. The plot and histogram are updated every 15 seconds. Figure 16.4 shows an example of a complete treatment on a large (6 × 6 × 3 cm) neck tumour. Two thermocouple arrays were placed in the tumour (a total of 10 junctions), one in the middle, about 1.5 cm deep, and the other near the base, about 2.5 cm deep. The temperature – time plots for array 1, situated about 1.5 cm deep in the tumour, are shown. Channel 1 was chosen to be the control thermocouple. The temperature rises up to about 42.5 °C and then levels out. In this case the target temperature was 43 °C but could not be reached because the power level had attained the maximum permitted by the program of 300 W. This limit, which may be changed, is incorporated in the program for safety reasons.

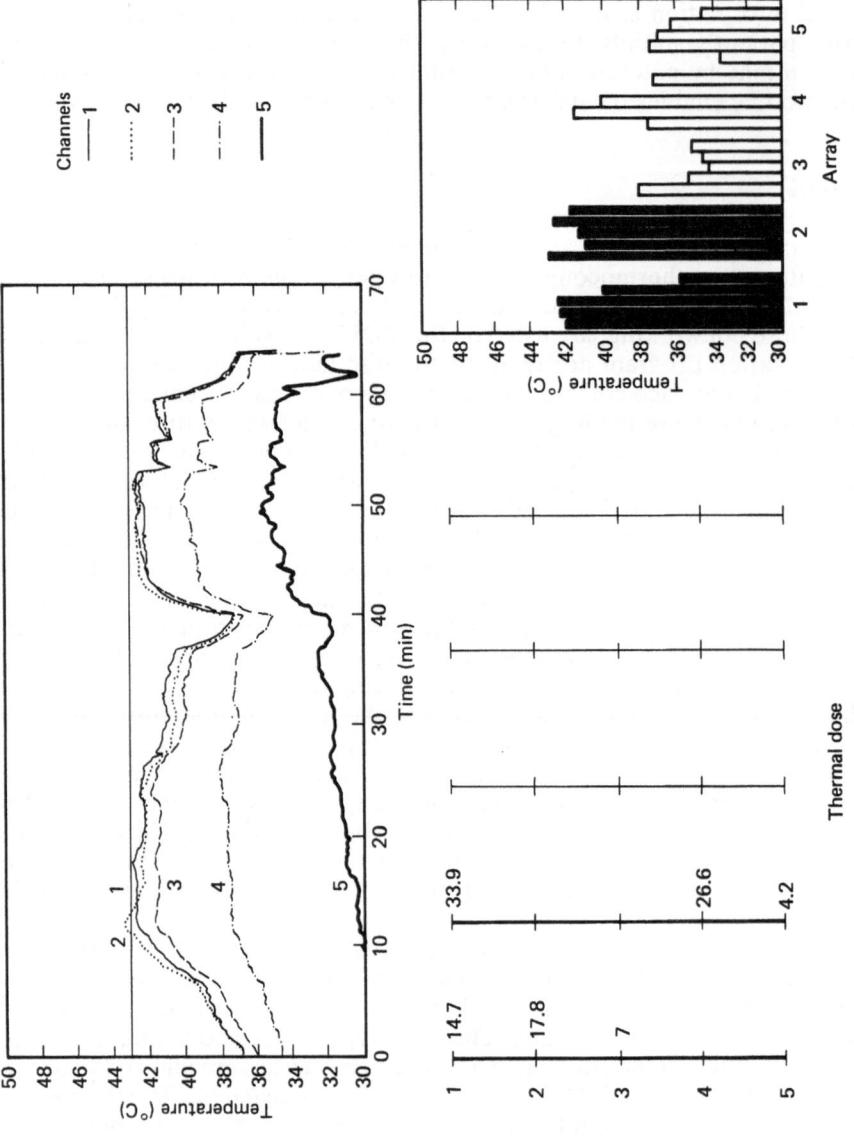

Fig. 16.4. Monitor display at the end of treatment. The fall in temperature in the middle of the treatment was due to the power being switched off while the position of the applicator was adjusted.

A very high power was required to heat this tumour, probably because a lot of heat was conducted away by the carotid artery lying beneath the tumour.

At the beginning of a 15-second cycle the power is switched off for 3 seconds to avoid errors due to electromagnetic pick-up and to allow the effects of any extra heating around the thermocouple junctions to decay. This can occur because the radio frequency field tends to concentrate around the metal thermocouple junctions. All 25 temperatures are measured in quick succession. If any of the thermocouples read more than two degrees over the target temperature the power is automatically switched off. After the 3 seconds of power off, the power is switched back on and the forward and reflected power measured. The forward power is that emitted by the radio frequency generator and fed into the applicator. The reflected energy is that not absorbed by the tumour and reflected back along the cable from the applicator. Normally only 10% or less of the forward power is reflected back, but this may increase if a matching problem develops, preventing optimum coupling of radio frequency power to the tumour. This sometimes happens if the patient moves.

Throughout the treatment the function keys are active (see Fig. 16.5). These enable the following tasks to be carried out:

1. Change the array plotted
2. Change the target temperature
3. Change the control thermocouple
4. Reduce the power immediately by 10% (patient too hot)
5. Vary the maximum power limit
6. Rescale graph

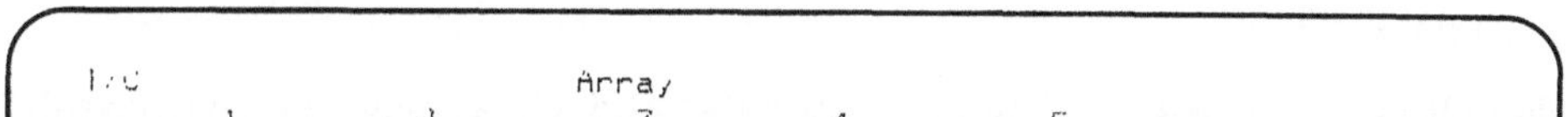

Fig. 16.5. VDU display during treatment.

  7. Power on/off
  8. Change heating rate or feedback control factor
  9. Switch between manual and automatic control
 10. Terminate

A control algorithm raises the temperature of a specified point in the tumour and maintains it at the target temperature. The algorithm has two sections, a boost phase and a steady phase. The boost phase controls the rate of temperature rise up to the target temperature, and the steady phase maintains the temperature at the target temperature. The algorithm is of the proportional type, i.e. the control value is incremented or decremented by a value that is proportional to the difference between the target temperature and the measured temperature. Each new control value is averaged with a number (usually 4) of the previous control values. This helps to smooth out fluctuations in temperatures. The boost phase maintains the rate of increase of temperature at about 1 °C per minute. When the temperature is within 0.2 °C of the target, or greater, the power is cut by a half and the steady phase algorithm is switched in. The temperature may be raised under manual control and the steady phase algorithm switched in when the temperature is fairly steady. Some patients are very sensitive to small increases in temperature (e.g. a change from 43 °C to 43.3 °C), and have different pain thresholds (some patients cannot tolerate much more than 41 °C). A control factor may be adjusted to reduce the response of the feedback loop.

Throughout the treatment, a quantity known as the thermal isoeffect dose (TID) is calculated. One thermal dose unit is defined as one minute at 43 °C (Dewey 1976; Field 1987; Sapareto and Dewey, 1984). The basic formula for calculating TID is:

$$TID = R^{T-43}$$

where $R = 2$ for $T > 42.5$ °C and $R = 6$ for $T < 42.5$ °C. As may be seen from this equation, 1 minute at 43 °C is equivalent to 30 seconds at 44 °C or 6 minutes at 42 °C. Five lines, divided into five, are drawn below the temperature–time plot (see Fig. 16.6). Each position on the lines represents a thermocouple junction. The top point represents the junction at the end of the array. The cumulative thermal dose at each junction is displayed in the appropriate position.

The treatment lasts for about 75 minutes in total, which is made up of a warm-up time of about 10 minutes, 60 minutes at 43 °C, and 5 minutes cooling off. The cooling curves can give information about the power absorption rate in the tumour and tumour blood flow.

Review

A program recalls the data and displays it in the same way that it appeared during treatment. A cursor may be moved across the temperature–time plot and the temperature and power values are displayed on the VDU. The histogram also plots the temperatures at the cursor position. A summary report is produced for each treatment. This is produced by the plotter on an A4 sheet of paper. An example is shown in Fig. 16.6. The temperature data are from a real treatment but the patient details have been changed.

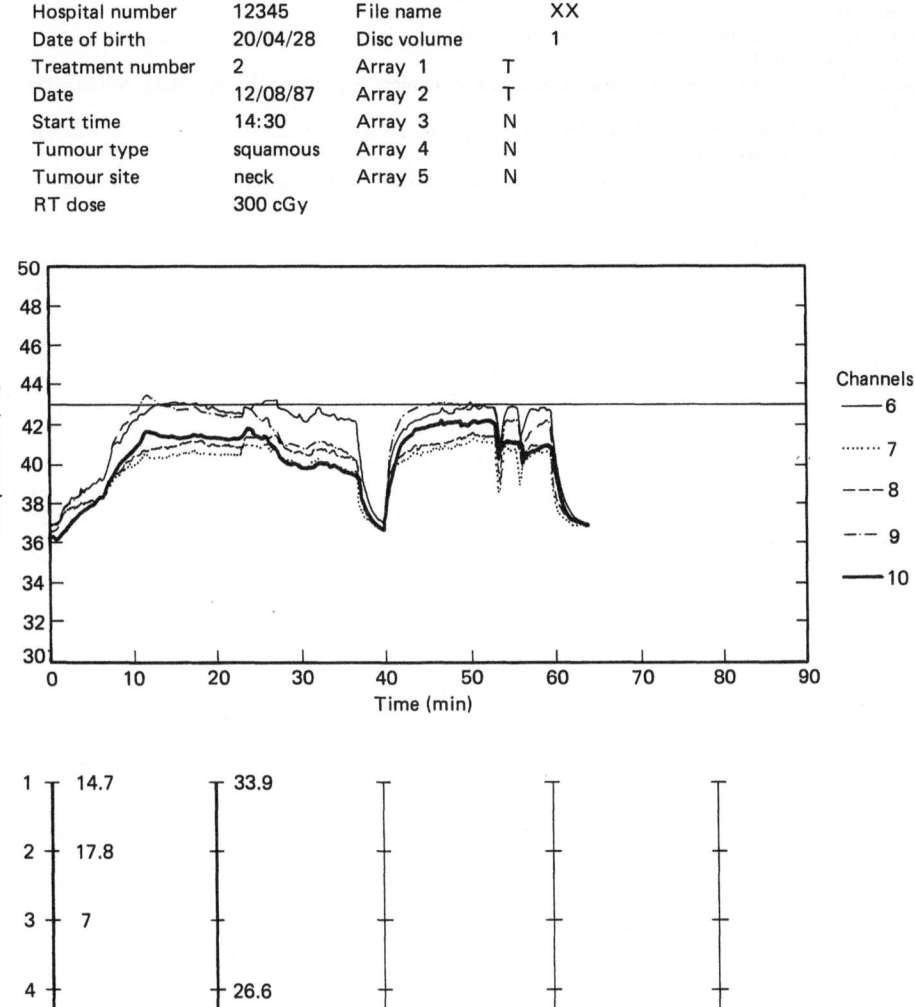

Patient name	A Patient	RT–HT interval	30 minutes
Hospital number	12345	File name	XX
Date of birth	20/04/28	Disc volume	1
Treatment number	2	Array 1	T
Date	12/08/87	Array 2	T
Start time	14:30	Array 3	N
Tumour type	squamous	Array 4	N
Tumour site	neck	Array 5	N
RT dose	300 cGy		

Fig. 16.6. Example of a summary report of a treatment.

References

Arcangeli G. (1983) Tumour control and therapeutic gain with different schedules of combined radiotherapy and local hyperthermia in human cancer. Int J Radiat Oncol Biol Phys 9: 1125–34

Coley WB, (1896) The therapeutic value of the mixed toxins of erysipelas and *Bacillus prodigeosus* in the treatment of inoperable malignant tumours. Am J Med Sci 112: 251–281

Conner WG (1977) Prospects for hyperthermia in human cancer therapy. II. Implications of biological and physical data for applications of hyperthermia in man. Radiology 123: 497–503

Dewey WC (1976) Cellular responses to combinations of hyperthermia and radiation. Radiology 123: 463–74

Field SB (1987) Studies relevant to a means of quantifying the effects of hyperthermia. Int J Hyperthermia 4: 291–296

Hand JW, James JR (1986) Physical techniques in clinical hyperthermia. Research Studies Press, Letchworth, England.

Sapareto SA, Dewey WC (1984) Thermal dose determination in cancer therapy. Int J Radiat Oncol Biol Phys 10: 787–800

Westermark N (1927) The effect of heat upon rat tumours. Skand Arch Physiol 52: 257–322

17 A Dermatological Advice System for Non-Experts

R.E. Ashton, G.J. Brooks and R. Pethybridge

Introduction

Family practitioners, service medical officers and paramedical staff often have to diagnose and treat skin disorders. Many find the task difficult because of the limited amount of dermatology experience included within their professional training programmes. Text books, packed with colour photographs, have long been available as a source of guidance. Unfortunately, although these may be useful for training, they cannot normally be used during consultations. A search of the photographs and chapters that contained information about the observed features of the patient's condition would be time-consuming, and would require some knowledge of the possible diagnosis.

Although computers have no inherent intelligence, their numerical and rapid data search attributes can benefit the user, if the computer has been efficiently programmed. A prototype suite of programs named DERMIS has been written in order to assist non-specialists with the diagnosis and management of common skin disorders. The diagnostic advice program has been designed to supplement human capabilities by providing a means of rapidly searching a disease database in order to detect similarities with the clinical findings.

When attempting the construction of such a search routine, decisions about technique have to be made. Most dermatological descriptors such as "papule" or "erythema" occur in many diseases with varying frequencies. Textbooks give some information on frequencies of clinical signs, and offer subjective opinion where frequencies are unknown. The simplest advice method would be for the computer to give a list of all the diseases that had any of the clinical features discovered on examination. Unfortunately, unordered listings produced by this method are long and not of much diagnostic value. A slight improvement can be made by eliminating from the list diseases that never present with the features found in the patient being investigated. Of more value to the user is a differential listing that has been placed in order of likelihood. To enable a program to achieve this, weightings must be assigned to the history and examination features.

A review of attempts to produce diagnostic programs in dermatology is given by Stoecker (1986). Haberman et al. (1985) used dermatologists to assign weightings to the features of diseases with which they were most familiar. These values were incorporated into a diagnostic program as a series of expert rules. The approach did not prove to be entirely successful as it was found that the estimated weightings often produced entirely the wrong result. The problem was tackled by using information from the cases that failed in order to modify the diagnostic rules.

Methods

In constructing DERMIS an attempt has been made to find the true frequencies of occurrence of various dermatological disease descriptors. This has been done by prospective case collection. Initially a dermatology case collection sheet was designed which incorporated all of the descriptive terms commonly used by dermatologists. Each term was defined and tested and all case information was collected according to the definitions.

The prospective database includes case details from patients presenting to the dermatology clinics at the Royal Naval Hospitals Haslar and Plymouth during the period 1985–1987. Information from each case was stored on computer and given a diagnostic label. The diagnosis had been established either at the time of consultation clinically or in the light of mycological or histological findings.

A diagnostic program was written using the first 2548 cases that had been collected. The cases on file were split into 32 disease groups, 31 of which made up 79% of the total. In determining the groups the dermatologist used individual diagnoses where either the number of cases in a diagnostic group was greater than about 20 or the diagnosis was considered important enough to be included separately. Some smaller diagnostic groups were combined where features and treatment were similar. Those not falling into any of the 31 main groups were combined and labelled REM or remainder. This last group (No. 32) is composed of a variety of cases of rarer disease that did not fit easily into any of the other groups. For each of the 32 groups the frequency of occurrence of the clinical features collected on the data sheet were calculated and used as weighting in the program. A relative likelihood algorithm was incorporated to provide some means of scoring each disease against new case information. From this a differential listing could be produced.

The prototype DERMIS program was written in MICROSOFT BASIC for use on an Apricot XI personal computer.

Results and Discussion

The prototype program was tested against data from a further 386 cases that had not been included in the database. The result of this analysis is given in

Table 17.1. The database size, number of cases tested during validation (showing number of cases correctly diagnosed with diagnostic failures itemised) are given for the diagnostic groups recognised

Diagnosis		Group size	Test number	Number correct	Computer prediction if diagnosis wrong
Alopecia areata	(AAR)	23	2	2	
Acne	(ACV)	133	21	21	
Basal cell carcinoma	(BCC)	143	28	27	NSP
Seborrhoeic wart	(BCP)	112	3	2	NCP
Solar keratosis	(SKE)	139	19	15	NID 2SCC REM
Epidermoid cyst	(CYE)	25	1	1	
Dermatofibroma	(DFM)	25	5	5	
Eczemas	(ECN)	371	59	46	6ECN 2LSC TCP 4REM
Hand and foot eczema	(ECE)	139	19	16	2TCP REM
Granuloma annulare	(GAN)	25	0		
Lentigo	(LEN)	15	4	4	
Lichen planus	(LPL)	31	4	4	
Lichen simplex	(LSC)	28	3	1	ECN ECE CYE WTV
Molluscum contagiosum	(MCN)	25	5	3	
Malignant melanoma	(MMN)	19	0		
Compound naevus	(NCP)	56	5	2	2NID NJN
Intradermal naevus	(NID)	50	13	5	2BCP CYE DFM MCN 3NCP
Junctional naevus	(NJN)	19	7	5	MMN NCP
Spider naevus	(NSP)	23	1	1	
Pyogenic granuloma	(PGR)	20	4	3	SCC
Psoriasis (plaque)	(PSP)	242	39	31	AAR 6ECA LSC
hands and feet	(PSE)	8	0		
hands pustular	(PPP)	19	1	1	
Pityriasis versicolor	(PVR)	33	7	5	NJN REM
Rosacea	(ROS)	24	4	3	REM
Squamous cell carcinoma	(SCC)	15	2		SKE
Skin tags	(STG)	19	2		2NID
Tinea	(TCP)	31	8	8	
Urticaria	(URT)	38	3	3	
Warts	(WTV)	122	32	23	4BCP 2NID NJN STG REM
Verruca	(WTS)	29	2	2	
Remainder	(REM)	537	80	20	ACE 5BCC 2BCP SKE CYE 4ECE 24ECN 4LPL 8LSC NID 2NJN NSP PGR PSG PVR 4SCC STG 2TCP WTV WTS
Overall diagnostic accuracy			255/386 = 66.1%		
Overall diagnostic accuracy excluding REM group			245/306 = 80%		

Table 17.1. The numbers of cases for each diagnostic group in the database and test series are listed in columns 3 and 4 respectively. In column 5 the number of cases where the correct diagnosis appeared first in the computer's differential list are given. Where diagnostic failure occurred, the computer's prediction is shown in the final column. Accuracy rates varied between groups but did not appear to depend directly on database group size.

The group that caused the most failures was the REM group which is composed of small numbers of cases of dissimilar diseases. None of these diseases can be accurately represented by frequency calculation as the features occurring commonly in one may be balanced by an uncommon occurrence of the same features in others. Predictably the majority of REM failures were of a false-negative type where the rare disease was diagnosed as belonging to one of the other 31 groups. If the failures from this REM group are excluded, the diagnostic accuracy of the program is increased to 77%. Other failures followed a predictable pattern between groups. Only diseases with similar features were confused with one another. This means that an appropriate differential listing is produced even if the first-appearing diagnosis is incorrect. The disease combinations used to produce the 32 groups have been reviewed in the light of the system's diagnostic errors. Reclassification of diseases into 42 groups has increased the overall diagnostic accuracy to 81% (paper submitted for publication).

It has been suggested that textbooks may not provide an easy source of diagnostic advice because of the time taken to shift for relevant information. In order to make best use of the rapid information access afforded by DERMIS, the computer interaction must be made as unobtrusive as possible. The final version of DERMIS may use a touch-sensitive device to capture patient information while the doctor is completing the data collection sheet. In this way, by the end of the consultation, computer advice will be available.

Dermatological Teaching Game

A dermatology teaching game has been devised that tests the user's knowledge against the frequency information contained in the database. A game flow-sheet is given in Fig. 17.1. Initially the computer selects a disease and the user is

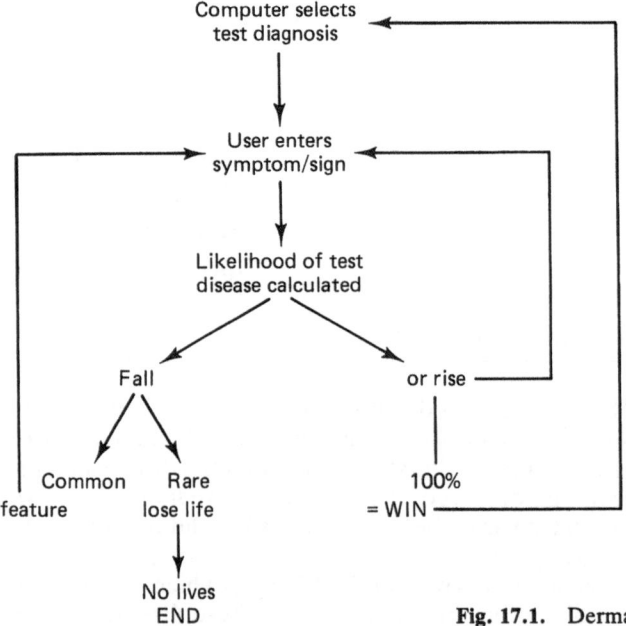

Fig. 17.1. Dermatology teaching game flow chart.

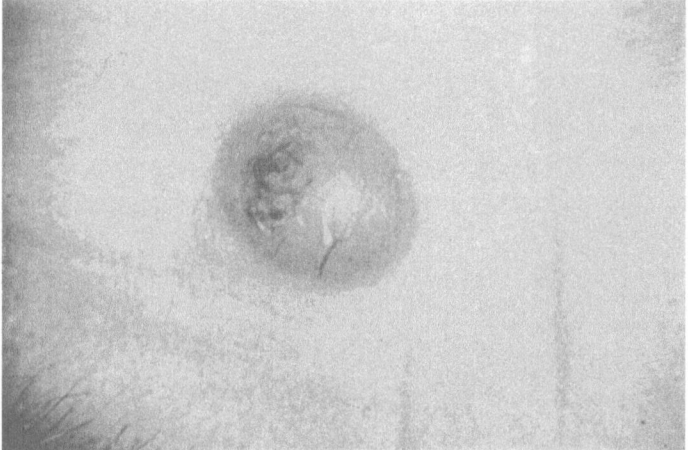

Fig. 17.2.   Clinical case for diagnosis: basal cell carcinoma.

requested to enter features that would support a diagnosis of that disease. If the player enters features that are uncommon and not predictive of the selected disease, then the computer subtracts a "life". The loss of all the player's "lives" ends the game and the computer then gives the player the option of listing the important features of the disease. If the computer assesses that the diagnosis has been confirmed, a score is calculated by dividing 100 by the number of features entered. This is added to the players total score, a "life" is gained and a new disease selected. It is hoped that, through playing the game, doctors, medical students and paramedical workers will be able to supplement their knowledge of the diagnostic features of common dermatological diseases.

Case Histories

The workings of the program are demonstrated on the three similar lesions shown in Figs. 17.2, 17.3 and 17.4, to give the reader some insight into how diagnoses are reached.

The essential clinical features that need to be identified for these lesions are listed in Table 17.2. If the features given are put into the program, the differential diagnoses shown in Table 17.3 are produced.

For Figs. 17.2 and 17.3, the diagnosis was not in doubt according to the computer, and agrees with the actual clinical diagnosis. In Fig 17.3, the first diagnosis is not so clearcut, and several alternatives are given in order of likelihood as calculated by the program. The correct diagnosis is the first one, an epidermoid cyst, but a dermatofibroma is possible.

To enable the reader to look into the workings of the program, Table 17.4 lists the frequencies for each of the clinical features for the diagnoses for Figs. 17.2, 17.3 and 17.4. In parentheses are listed the predictive factor of the sign/symptom for each diagnosis. This is calculated by taking the ratio (as a percentage) of the

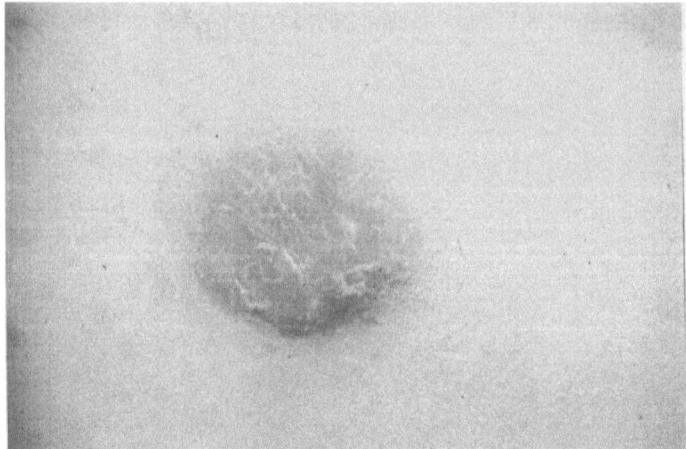

Fig. 17.3. Clinical case for diagnosis: dermatofibroma (histiocytoma).

Table 17.2. Essential clinical features to identify lesions shown in Figs. 17.2, 17.3 and 17.4

	Fig. 17.2	Fig. 17.3	Fig. 17.4
Age of patient	65 years	25 years	40 years
Lesion/rash	Single lesion	Single lesion	Single lesion
Site	Face	Leg	Trunk
Size	8 mm	10 mm	13 mm
Type[a]	Papule	Papule	Nodule
Colour	Pink	Pink-purple	Normal
Shape	Round	Round	Round
Border	Well defined	Well defined	Well defined
Surface	Normal and crust	Scaly	Normal
Palpation	Firm	Firm	Firm
Vascular features	Telangiectasia	None	None

[a] Nodule: raised rounded lesions greater than 1 cm in diameter.
Papule: raised lesion less than 1 cm in diameter.

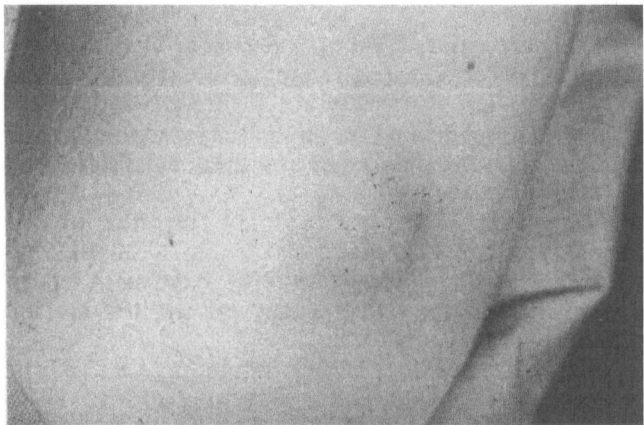

Fig. 17.4. Clinical case for diagnosis: epidermoid (sebaceous) cyst.

Table 17.3. Differential diagnoses for lesions shown in Figs. 17.2, 17.3 and 17.4

Fig. 17.2	Basal cell carcinoma	100%[a]
Fig. 17.3	Dermatofibroma	99%[a]
	Lichen planus	1%
Fig. 17.4	Epidermoid (sebaceous) cyst	61%[a]
	Dermatofibroma	33%
	Viral warts	2%
	Compound naevus	1%
	Pyogenic granuloma	1%

[a] Computer generated relative likelihood score, calculated by the equation $R(D^1/S) = P(S/D^1)/P(S/D)$ where $R(D^1/S)$ is the relative likelihood of disease D^1 given the particular set of symptoms and signs (S), $P(S/D^1)$ is the probability of the particular set of symptoms and signs in disease D^1, $P(S/D)$ is the summation of the probability of the set of symptoms and signs for all possible diseases D.

Table 17.4. Computer-generated relative likelihood scores and predictive factors of the clinical features of the diagnoses for the lesions illustrated in Figs. 17.2, 17.3 and 17.4

Clinical feature				Diagnosis					
	Basal cell carcinoma			Dermatofibroma			Epidermoid cyst		
	Fig. 17.2	freq	factor	Fig. 17.3	freq	factor	Fig. 17.4	freq	factor
Age	[65 years]	25	(7)	[40 years]	19	(4)	[25 years]	32	(5)
Single lesion		90	(8)		68	(6)		63	(6)
Site	[face]	73	(7)	[arm]	68	(10)	[arm]	32	(4)
Type of lesion	[papule]	43	(4)	[papule]	84	(6)	[nodule]	74	(24)
Colour	[pink]	62	(5)	[pink-purple]	16	(5)	[normal]	84	(15)
Shape round		50	(4)		94	(8)		95	(8)
Border well defined		73	(4)		90	(4)		95	(5)
Surface	[crust]	50	(18)	[scale]	16	(2)	[normal]	99	(6)
Palpation firm		40	(6)		77	(11)		84	(12)
Telangiectasia		33	(14)		0			0	

frequency of a sign (or symptom) for a diagnosis to the summation of frequencies of same sign for all diagnoses.

A factor with a high value indicates that the symptom in question is an important one in distinguishing this diagnosis from all other. For example, telangiectasia in basal cell carcinoma has a factor of 14 but only occurs in 33% of patients with a basal cell carcinoma. On the other hand, 90% of basal cell carcinoma (recorded in the database) are single but the predictive factor for this feature is only 8 since many other types of lesion occur singly. Epidermoid cysts are nodules in 74% of cases, and since few other types of lesion (within the database) are nodular, this feature has a high predictive factor (24).

If the features for Fig. 17.3 are changed so that papule (i.e. less than 1 cm in size) replaces nodule, then the diagnostic list (with relative likelihood scores) becomes:

Dermatofibroma (67%)

Viral warts (10%)

Skin tags (9%)

Epidermoid cyst (4%)

Table 17.5. Computer-generated relative likelihood scores and diagnoses predicted as clinical features for Fig. 17.2 added to preceding ones successively.

Clinical feature	BCC	SKE	NID	Diagnosis predicted[a] BCP	CYE	LEN	NSP	MMN
Age 65 years		8		8		10		8
+ single lesion	15	11		11		19		15
+ face	22	12			12	24	9	
+ papule	23	18	12	10	11			
+ pink	40	24	13	5			9	
+ round	44	9	28	5	9			
+ crust	92	6	0	1				
+ firm	96	2		1				
+ telangiectasia	100							

[a] BCC = Basal cell carcinoma
SKE = Solar keratosis
NID = Intradermal melanocytic naevus (mole)
BCP = Basal cell papilloma (seborrhoeic wart)
CYE = Cyst epidermoid (sebaceous cyst)
LEN = Lentigo (liver spot)
NSP = Spider naevus
MMN = Malignant melanoma

If the program were accompanied by descriptive features and, possibly, by photographs of each of these lesions, it should be possible clinically to eliminate viral warts, skin tags and possibly dermatofibroma, again achieving the correct diagnosis of epidermoid cyst.

Another way of looking into the workings of the program is to examine the changes in diagnosis as each clinical feature is added on. The features for Fig. 17.2 are put into the program in sequence (i.e. "age 65" entered first, followed by "single lesion" etc.) and the relative likelihood score as each feature is added for diagnoses is shown in Table 17.5. Initially lentigo (a flat brown patch) is the most likely diagnosis until papule is entered. Lentigo then falls out of the differential since (by definition) these lesions are never raised (papular). Basal cell carcinoma now is the most likely diagnosis, and as the features are entered this possibility increases to eventually 100%. The second most likely diagnosis is a solar keratosis (rough scaly papule or plaque on the face of older people due to chronic sun exposure). It is of interest that the computer's differential list becomes shorter as more features are added.

Conclusion

The development of the DERMIS diagnostic advice and teaching programs is not complete. The database is continually being updated and the methods of using it improved by the inclusion of new techniques. In the near future a fully operational version of the system will be available for use by family practitioners and paramedical staff. The program is not intended for specialist dermatologists as the system provides advice only for conditions commonly referred to specialists.

Summary

A diagnostic and teaching aid for common skin disorders, named DERMIS, is described. The program uses a database derived from the prospective collection of 2548 cases seen in a routine dermatological clinic. These were divided into 32 diagnostic groups. The system uses a relative likelihood algorithm. The computer placed the correct diagnosis first in the differential list in 66% of 386 further cases tested. The workings of the diagnostic program are illustrated by reference to three similar cases, and the use of the database to produce a dermatological teaching game is described.

Acknowledgements. The authors would like to thank Janssen Pharmaceutical Ltd for their financial assistance.

References

Haberman HF, Norwich KH, Diehl DL et al. (1985) DIAG: A computer-assisted dermatologic diagnostic system – clinical experience and insight. J Am Acad Dermatol 1: 132–143
Stoecker WV (1986) Computer-aided diagnosis of dermatologic disorders. Dermatol Clin 4: 607–625

18 Computerised Management of Sterile Supplies

R.J. Whiddett

Introduction

This chapter has two main themes: its primary focus is the description of the development and implementation of a computerised multi-user system for managing the operation of a sterile supplies department; its secondary focus is to illustrate how the features of the Pick Operating System are well suited to solving these sorts of problems. A more complete introduction to the use of Pick is given in the book by Bull (1987).

Operation of Sterile Supplies Departments

The sterile supplies departments are among the many unsung heros of the National Health Service. Every day, the smooth passage of the vast numbers of patients who pass through the NHS is crucially dependent on copious supplies of a wide range of sterile instruments and dressing packs being available whenever they are needed. The central sterile supplies departments (CSSD) are usually responsible for the needs of a whole health service district, sometimes with the aid of several smaller theatre sterile supplies units (TSSU) which provide a dedicated service to small groups of operating theatres.

A CSSD is a small factory which assembles collections of surgical instruments and dressings and sterilises them to form a "sterile pack". The scale of operation and the range of products produced by a CSSD is quite remarkable. Typically 1000 different types of items may be used in the assembly of packs, and these range from cotton-wool balls which cost virtually nothing, to precision surgical instruments which cost tens or hundreds of pounds each. The CSSD manager must keep adequate stocks of each of these items to meet the demands to manufacture packs. They are assembled in many different combinations to form hundreds of different sterile packs. The composition of some packs may be trivially simple; for example, a pair of scissors in a plastic bag; others, such as a tray of theatre instruments, may contain tens or even hundreds of items. A district CSSD may well be serving over 100 different locations, which may require over 10 000 packs per week between them. Some packs contain only disposable items, such as swabs and dressings, which are discarded after use. Others also contain some instruments that may be reused, in which case the instruments are returned to the CSSD where they are inspected, repaired if necessary, repacked and sterilised. Eventually, most items become too worn to repair and are replaced.

Historically, the CSSD owned all the instruments and was provided with an adequate annual budget to cover running expenses, the purchase of additional or replacement instruments, and to pay for the disposable dressings. The recent years of financial stringency within the NHS have caused CSSD managers to seek greater control over the use of their resources and to instil a degree of cost-consciousness amongst their clients, by keeping detailed records of the use of resources.

With the proposed introduction of management budgeting, CSSD will effectively lose its budget and will have to recoup its expenses by presenting its clients with detailed, realistic charges for the use of packs. In the future, a CSSD management information system will have to be tailored specifically to the application, to be very efficient to use, and interface directly to the NHS standard accounting systems, such as SAS. Such a system has now been implemented at the Sterile Supplies Department at Bath.

Computer System Overview

The operation of a sterile supplies department is an extension of that of a normal health services central stores operation, so it is logical to implement a sterile supplies management system as an extension to a stores information system. The system was developed from the Wessex Enhanced Stores Information System (WESSIS) (WESSIS Users Manual 1986), a multi-user system which runs on microcomputers under the Pick Operating System. WESSIS provides a comprehensive stock control system; it consists of approximately 150 program modules which record the ordering, delivery, invoicing, payment and despatch of general stock items and of special items which are not usually held as stock in a depot. WESSIS records all transactions and can respond to an extensive range of on-line enquiries concerning individual items or groups of items; it also provides extensive management and financial reports and an interface to the accounting system SAS.

An overview of the CSSD management system is given in Fig. 18.1. The WESSIS system provides the framework for the entire system, and also provides the stock control of the store of non-sterile items. The program modules which perform the stock control and issuing of sterilising packs are based extensively on the standard stock system, but many new programs had to be produced to deal with the return of used instruments and the manufacture of packs from their components.

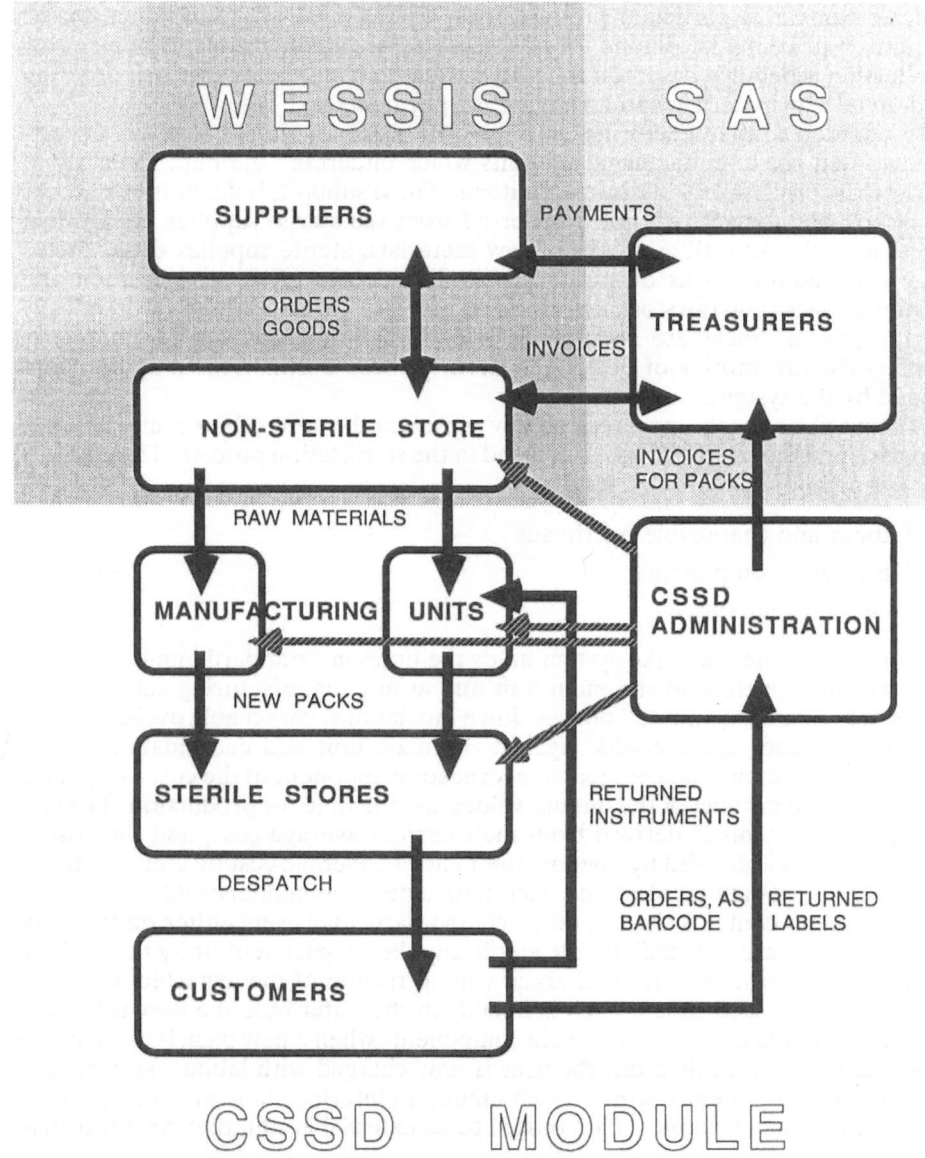

Fig. 18.1. An overview of the CSSD management system.

Overview Of The Software Modules

The management of a sterile supplies department can be likened to that of a small firm. The customers, i.e. wards and theatres, send in orders on a regular basis. The orders are filled and despatched and the client is sent regular statements of accounts. It differs from the small firm in that each of the customers is allocated a specific number of particular product lines, and as these are used the customer requires replacements. Behind the scenes, there are all the problems of planning production schedules based on the anticipated demand, stock control, ordering additional raw materials and arranging for payment.

In addition to manufacturing on their own premises, sterile supplies departments often use manufacturing subunits which undertake the bulk assembly of packs that consist solely of disposable items. These subunits hold their own stocks of disposable items which are transferred from the sterile supplies department general stock. As well as stocks of raw materials, sterile supplies departments may keep buffer stocks of sterile packs. The details of the composition and costing of packs and the stock level in the buffer stock is maintained automatically by the system. Packs are also stored prior to use in wards and in emergency cupboards. Inventories of packs allocated to these destinations may be maintained by the system.

The pricing of packs must realistically represent the costs of the components of the pack and the overhead costs incurred in the sterilisation process. The cost of a pack is composed of three parts:

1. Labour and chargeable overheads
2. Disposable components
3. Reusable components

For each sterile pack, the system holds the times in "standard minutes" that it takes to manufacture at the main unit and at any manufacturing subunit. The costs of a "standard minute" broken down into labour, chargeable overheads and estate overheads are recorded against the main unit and each manufacturing subunit. The labour and chargeable overheads component of the cost of a pack is derived as the product of the minute values and the time for production. The cost of disposable items is derived from their current average cost, and the cost of reusable items is derived by dividing their current average cost by their estimated life. These costs are recalculated each time a pack is manufactured.

The system contains the option to charge particular users either on the basis that the packs are "owned" by the sterile supplies department or by themselves. In the former case the user is charged with a fraction of the expected life of the reusable items each time a pack is issued. In the latter case the user is initially charged with the cost of the reusable components when a new pack is made up for the first time. From then on, the user is only charged with labour, service, and disposable component charges. Each month an interface tape may be produced which allows issue charges to be passed to an external accounting system such as SAS.

The system requires that the manufacture, issue, and return or use of all packs be recorded. To cope with this extensive demand for information, bar-coded labels and bar-code readers may be used to record these movements. However, the use of bar codes is not essential, as the data may be manually entered via a terminal keyboard. The details of bar-code devices is covered in a later section.

After use, the reusable instruments from packs are returned to the sterile supplies department, together with either the bar-coded labels from all packs (including those containing only disposable components) or a hand-written requisition for replacements. If bar-coded labels are in use it is assumed that a replacement pack is required for each returned label. If a pack originates from an emergency cupboard, a replacement is despatched to the cupboard, but its cost is charged to the user.

After the recording of the return/use of packs the following three reports may be produced:

1. A checklist of the reusable items which should have been returned from each customer
2. A consolidated manufacturing schedule for the replacement packs
3. A despatch list of the replacement packs for each customer

These reports need not all be produced at the same time; the production of each of them may be fitted into the schedule of the department. The checklist (item 1), details all the instruments that should have been returned from each customer; if items are missing or damaged then replacements will have to be issued from stock. The consolidated manufacturing list (item 2), details the replacement packs to be manufactured. The program has options to produce a bulk picking list for the disposable components, and bar-coded labels for the packs. Once the packs have been manufactured they are booked into the sterile store, again using bar-coded labels. This operation automatically records the issue of the disposable components from the appropriate main and subunit component stores. Care should be taken that all component stocks are booked into the components store before the manufacture of packs that require them are recorded: the system will not allow the component stock to become negative as this is both illogical, and leads to nonsensical pricing of components. Similarly, if buffer stocks of sterile packs are limited or non-existent, it will be necessary to record their manufacture before they can be issued. The despatch list (item 3) details the replacement packs to be despatched to each customer. Once these packs have been assembled they may be recorded as issued.

As with the standard stock system, transactions concerning the stock level or value of the sterile stocks are logged in a file which provides a full audit trail. To aid the planning of production, the system may keep detailed histories of the quantities of each pack that are issued to each transfer point each month, from which graphic displays and printed reports can be produced.

The Selection of the Hardware

To minimise implementation costs, the system was installed as a separate account on a large General Automation (GA) Zebra processor which was already running in the stores department on Chippenham. This machine is accessed from Bath over leased telephone lines. However, it was developed on much smaller systems and should perform satisfactorily on a small system with a 30 Mbyte Winchester disc.

The selection of bar-coding hardware aimed at gaining the greatest flexibility in the use of equipment and providing the greatest potential for expansion within the constraints of the following system requirements:

1. To be able to produce bar-coded labels for products using NSV coding, i.e. including alphabetic characters.

2. To give an initial daily rate of production of 1000 labels per day; these need to be produced rapidly to avoid delaying the production of the day's work, so the maximum printing time needs to be about 1 hour.

3. Bar codes need to be conveniently read on-line when returned goods are unpacked and checked, so full screen display or local hardcopy device is required.

4. The system had to run on GA Zebra hardware under the Pick operating system.

Bar-Coding

There is a plethora of bar-code systems. The requirement to represent alphabetic characters restricts the choice to the emerging standard CODE 39, (also known as 3 of 9), or the less widely available Telepen code. CODE 39 was chosen as it offers the widest choice of hardware.

The system is of small size and does not warrant the use of extensive bar-code networking and concentrating systems of the form intended for major factories so interfaces to standard serial lines were adequate. There are three choices of hardware architecture for on-line readers: stand-alone reader stations; "wedges" that interface between the keyboard and the monitor unit of a terminal and translate the bar codes into the signals that the equivalent keys would produce; "wedges" that interface on the serial line between the terminal and the processor and translate the bar-codes into the equivalent character codes which are transmitted to the processor.

Stand-alone stations tend to have restricted display capabilities and therefore were unsuitable for the interactive receiving of goods in this application and keyboard wedges were not appropriate as they are usually restricted to use with a particular terminal type, so a serial line interface was chosen. Since this unit has to interface directly to the processor it was essential that it produced ASCII codes and supported the XON/XOFF flow control protocol used by GA, not the more common hardware RTS/CTS protocol. The latter constraint proved quite difficult to satisfy. Our initial choice of hardware was a new product, but it showed intermittent timing problems and occasionally lost data which suggested that there were problems in the implementation of the flow control. Finally, we chose more mature equipment from Intermec, which has proved very reliable.

Bar-coded labels may be produced in three ways: by using dedicated bar-code printers, laser printers with suitable font cartridges or special purpose matrix printers. Each of these types of machines recognise an escape sequence which puts them into bar-code printing mode, and they perform the translation automatically from the ASCII code to the printed bar code.

The relatively small quantity of labels to be produced did not warrant the use of a dedicated printer. With a label size of approximately 4" × 1", laser printers could produce 1000 labels in about 10 minutes. However, there are reservations concerning the use of labels with automatic sheet feeders, and manual feeding of labels may reduce the actual throughput considerably. A high speed matrix printer, (ca 250 cps), can produce the 1000 labels required in approximately 1 hour, which was fast enough for our purposes. Our initial choice was to use a third-party card interfacing to a fast Epson printer, but we encountered problems in maintaining the alignment between the printer and the labels. Our final choice has been a Mannesmann Tally MT460D printer which has a built-in bar-coding feature; this has proved very satisfactory, and with a discount it was only about 30% more expensive than the Epson.

The Pick Operating System

The origins of Pick can be traced back to the mid 1960s, when its concepts were developed as a database system; then in the 1970s it was extended to act as a complete stand-alone multi-user operating system. The techniques used in the design of Pick mean that it is relatively easy to implement on new machines, and it is now widely available on microprocessor-based systems. It is popular because it is a true multi-user system, designed to allow the safe and coordinated sharing of data using the concept of locking individual records within files, and because of the advantages of its unique method of implementing files. Other multi-user features include the sharing of peripheral devices under the control of a spooler, an accounting system to record the utilisation of resources and some security features to restrict the capabilities of users. Common application programs, such as word processors and spread sheets, are also available but they tend not to be quite as sophisticated as those found on single-user micros.

Pick's unusual origins in a "data-oriented" environment and its particular file structure give it a significantly different "feel" from "process-oriented" systems such as Unix and MS–DOS, and the organisation of Pick's file system is less secure than that of the latter systems. However, this insecurity can be controlled if the application programs are implemented as a "turnkey" system which never allows the users to gain direct access to the operating system. WESSIS and the CSSD module were developed in this way using the programming tools of APT (APT Utilities Manual 1986). One APT tool generates a menu system with an integrated security system that restricts the programs that a user can access. Another useful feature provided by APT is a set of standard keyboard routines which can be used in application programs to provide a consistent user interface. The routines simplify the programming of program interruptions, the provision of default input values and the validation of input.

The most striking feature of Pick is the unique structure of its files. Files consist of set of records (called items in Pick terminology) which are identified within the file by a unique key value, which is used by the hashing algorithms when the item is stored or retrieved. Items cannot be considered to be ordered within the file; any specific ordering of items must be imposed by explicitly programming an index to the file.

The items within a file may vary in structure and size; they consist of a series of attributes, which may be subdivided into a series of values, which again may be divided into a series of subvalues. Each of these components may be of any size provided that the total size of the item remains less than 32 kbytes. Unlike more traditional database systems, which use a fixed record size and "pad-out" fields which are shorter than the maximum length, Pick explicitly indentifies the end of each component of an item with special characters and the item expands or contracts as components change their size. All the details of these operations are hidden from the user and even the programmer, since the programming language provided with Pick systems is an extended BASIC which includes standard routines to unpack items into their components when they are read from a file and to repack them when they are written back to the file. Another useful feature of the language is that it automatically coerces data variables into the appropriate form (i.e. numeric or character strings) when they are accessed.

The benefits of Pick's flexible file structure are illustrated by the following simplified example of an item in the file which contains the information concerning sterile packs:

Key:	NSV Code:	PAK001		
Attribute 1:	Name:	General Pack		
Attribute 2:	Group:	gen		
Attribute 3:	Quantity:	254		
Attribute 4:	Value:	623		
. . .				
. . .				
Attribute 19:	Components:	cwb001]swa001]	. . . . . .]	sca002
Attribute 20:	Qty:	12] 6]	. . . . . .]	3

Each type of pack is identified by a unique NSV (National Standard Vocabulary) code, which can be used to identify its item in the PACKS file. Each item then consists of a number of attributes which are used to store information about packs of this form; in practice there are 20 attributes containing the pack's name, product group, quanitity in stock, value of stock, date when last manufactured etc.

The meaning of the information held in an attribute is determined solely by the interpretation imposed upon it by the programs that manipulate it, and it is the responsibility of the programmer to ensure the consistent interpretation of information. The flexibility of the file structure means that it is not necessary to impose any restrictions on variable length attributes, such as the name of the pack, during the design of the file. In practice the programs which input and display attribute values usually impose some maximum size, but if these limits are changed they do not affect the file structure.

The two final attributes in the example illustrate the use of multiple values. Both attributes consist of a list of values separated by the value-mark character which is represented as]. The "components" attribute contains a list of codes identifying all the different types of components that are required to manufacture the particular pack. This list can be of whatever length is necessary to define the pack, and typically consists of between 2 and 50 items. The final attribute contains a multi-valued list which defines the quantity required for the corresponding element in the list of components. This scheme easily accommodates the wide range in the complexity of the composition of packs.

In addition to the data stored in a Pick file, there is also an associated dictionary which can be used to define the format of the information contained within the file. These dictionary terms may be used within commands expressed in a high-level, forth-generation language, called ACCESS (ACCESS Reference Manual 1984) or ENGLISH which is supplied with Pick systems. ACCESS commands can be used to construct ad-hoc enquiries directly from a user's terminal or they may be issued from within a BASIC program to produce sophisticated reports. A dictionary item defines the way in which a piece of information can be derived from the information within the file, and the way in which the result is to be presented. For example, a dictionary item called NAME could be associated with the packs file which would indicate that the pack's name could be found in the first attribute and that it should be printed in reports in a field 25 characters wide. The simple ACCESS command SORT PACKS NAME would then produce a list of all the names of packs within the file sorted into alphabetical order. More sophisticated dictionary items can be used to select parts of attributes, apply format conversions and arithmetic operations, or to use the information to retrieve data from another file. Dictionary terms are difficult to define and should be set up by the programmer during the development of the system, but once defined they are easy to use.

The ACCESS language can easily be used to produce a wide range of reports using features to select subsections of a file, to produce subtotals and totals, or to handle multi-valued lists in a sensible way. The use of ACCESS commands within BASIC programs simplifies many of the more mundane aspects of program development and greatly enhances the productivity of programmers.

Summary

The development of the system began in autumn 1986 and involved the close cooperation of all the interested parties, including the CSSD manager and representatives from the treasurer's department. The facilities of the Pick Operating System's file organisation encourages the development of applications using prototyping techniques. This meant that modules could be evaluated by the users as they were developed and they were occasionally modified as the system evolved. The system has been in operation since spring 1987, and the users are very satisfied with it.

The selection of reliable bar-coding equipment proved more difficult than expected, but with satisfactory hardware the use of bar codes has proved so successful that their application has been extended to allow the input of other data, such as transfer point codes.

References

ACCESS Reference Manual (1984). General Automation Inc. Anahern, California
APT Utilities Manual (1986) Real Computer Systems. Wychbold, Worcestershire
Bull M (1987) The Pick Operating System. Chapman and Hall, London
WESSIS Users Manual (1986) Wessex Regional Health Authority, Winchester

19 A Computerised References Management System

A.M. Seifalian, R.L. Vaghjiani and K.E.F. Hobbs

Introduction

It is essential for a research department to develop a filing system which will allow easy and comprehensive indexing of scientific papers which are collected. The system must be capable of indexing, storing and retrieving information related to authors' names, title of the paper, journal in which it is published and a list of key words. One method is to record the citations on cards, another is to use a computer. There are several large mainframe-based bibliographic reference systems which include Medline and Excerpta Medica in the biomedical fields. These are usually based in major libraries and are very comprehensive but can only produce a reference to a published work and occasionally a summary. When the researcher obtains a copy of the paper, he needs to store it for future reference.

Hunter (1983) and Kunin (1985) described a computer program that allows the user to build and search through a library of collected scientific papers. We describe an extension and refinement of that program. Our goal was to design an easy-to-use, general-purpose system for indexing and filing stored scientific papers. Using our program we can search for a paper reference for a key word, author, part or whole of the title, or journal name. The selected references can be arranged alphabetically or in the house style of any selected journal.

Hardware

The size and model of computer will depend on the magnitude of the task set for it in terms of the number and size of the scientific papers to be stored, and the number of other computers linked into the system. We choose to use an IBM AT with 30 MByte Winchester disc because of its processing speed and its ability to be linked easily to other similar computers to form a local area network. This allows

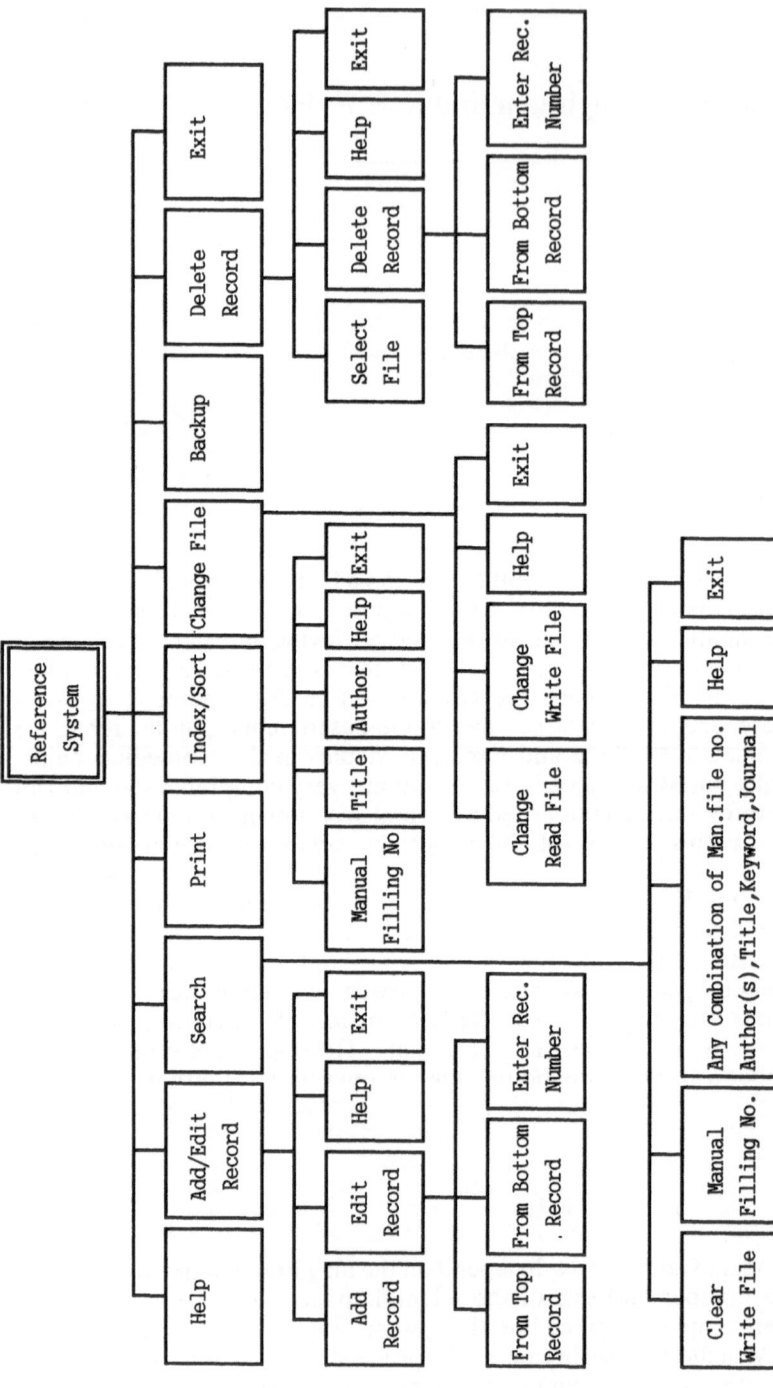

Fig. 19.1. Reference record system menu hierarchy.

a fast response time for data input, searches and data back-up even when the number of papers collected exceeds several thousand.

Software

The program is written in dBase III+ (Ashton Tate, Oaklands, 1 Bath Road, Maidenhead, Berks) fourth-generation language and WordStar 2000 (MicroPro International Ltd, Haygarth House, 28–31 High Street, Wimbledon Village, London SW19 5BY). dBase fourth-generation language was used because it is very similar to, but easier than the PASCAL programming language and encourages the use of structured programming methods. This is a program implementation technique that systematises and organises the entire cycle of program design, coding and testing. The ultimate goal of this technique is to develop correct reliable programs by preventing errors and facilitating debugging. Structured programming also attempts to develop software that minimises personal costs and increases productivity. Other advantages of the dBase III include in-built procedures such as sort, search and index which can be easily implemented in the program for fast and efficient responses. It enables the programmer to compile all the procedures into a compact, encoded form. The encoded procedures can then be linked into one program which increases execution speed. It can support local area networking (LAN) which we plan to implement shortly.

The dBase language is composed of three components:

1. Top-down design with stepwise refinements (Fig. 19.1)
2. Independent program modules
3. Structural coding principles

The primary purpose of components 2 and 3 is to provide highly readable and understandable programs for future development or modification. Figure 19.2 shows the segments of the program that handle operator interaction, disc file and record assignment. Each filed scientific paper has the following entries: manual filing number, author(s), title, journal, volume, pages, a list of key words and the potential for a summary of up to 5000 characters. Each record can later be modified or deleted in case of multiple entries.

The program can display the references on screen or they can be printed out, using one of many print formats provided. The system was developed to ensure that it was user friendly and to have a consistent layout of all menu screens, thus avoiding unnecessary confusion to the user. The functions available from the main menu screen (Fig. 19.3) are described below.

Help

The Reference System is based on a hierarchy of menus, each providing instructions. But a more extensive help function can be called at all stages in case of difficulty.

```
* Program : MAINmenu.prg
* Purpose : Reference System Main Menu.
*
* initialise system
DO Initiali
*
* main loop
DO WHILE .T.
    * display menu choices
    progtitl='Main  Menu'
    DO CLS_scrn
    DO MENUscrn
    *
    SET COLOR TO n/bg
    @ 13,33 SAY 'Please make a selection using a function key.'
    SET COLOR TO n/w
    key=0
    *
    DO WHILE key>=0 .and. key<>28
        key=INKEY()
        @ 22,69 SAY TIME()
    ENDDO
    @ 22,69 SAY '          '
    *
    DO CASE
        CASE key=F1
            DO Get_HELP WITH 'ALL'      && display all help pages
            *
        CASE key=-1
            DO EDIT_ref                 && edit old refs. or add new ones
            *
        CASE key=-2
            DO Search                   && search for references
            *
        CASE key=-3
            DO DELE_rec                 && allow deletion unwanted refs.
            *
        CASE key=-4
            DO Set_INDX                 && select a new index
            *
        CASE key=-5
            DO PRINTref                 && print refs. in required format
            *
        CASE key=-6
            DO ChngFILE                 && select a new current read file
            *
        CASE key=-7
            DO BACK_dbf                 && backup database files
            *
        CASE key=-8
            DO LOAD_dbf                 && reload backed up files
            *
        CASE key=F10
            DO EXIT_sys                 && exit from reference system
            *
    ENDCASE
ENDDO
RETURN
* eof: MAINmenu.prg
```

Fig. 19.2. Listing of main program and description of subroutines.

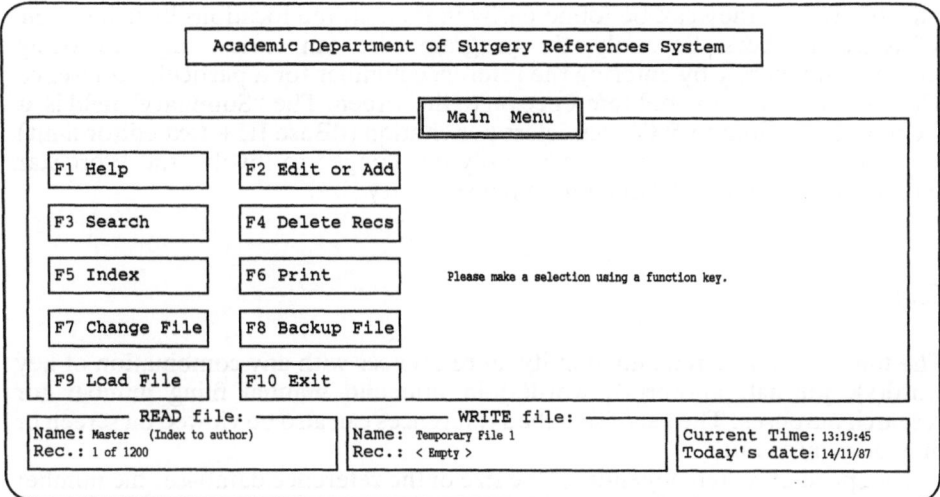

Fig. 19.3. Display of references system main menu.

Edit or Add

First, the user must select whether he wants to add new citations or edit previously entered ones. For editing, the user selects the appropriate citation, enters the editor screen shown in Fig. 19.4 and types in the amendment. The program also assigns a number to each reference entry. This number is useful in two ways. First, copies of the reprints can be filed in consecutive order according to these assigned numbers. Thus, when a search of the reference data base yields

```
 _____
|                                                                         |
|          Academic Department of Surgery References System               |
|                                                                         |
|                        _____                        |
|                       |     Edit  or  Add       |                       |
|    _____|                         |_____   |
|   |                      Manual Filing Number: [_____]             |  |
|   | Ctrl PgUP add to or                                              |  |
|   |      edit the summary.  Authors: [_____]  |
|   |      summary.                                                    |  |
|   |                         Title:   [_____]  |
|   | PgUp will move back                                              |  |
|   |      one record.        Journal: [_____]      |
|   | PgDn will move forward                                           |  |
|   |      one record.        Year: [___]  Volume: [_____]  Page(s): [__]|
|   |                                                                  |  |
|   | Esc  will bring you     Keyword(s): [_____]  |
|   |      back to the                                                 |  |
|   |      options menu.                                               |  |
|   |_____|  |
|    _____ READ file: _____      _____ WRITE file: _____              |
|   | Name: Master (Index to manual) | Name: Master        | Current Time: 13:19:45 |
|   | Rec.: 1202 of 1202             | Rec.: 1202 of 1202  | Today's date: 14/11/87 |
|_____|
```

Fig. 19.4. Display of add or edit menu.

a list of articles, they can be found easily in their stored locations by using their reference numbers. Secondly, the program user can review any previously entered data merely by entering the reference number for a particular reference which will call back the full reference on to the screen. The "Summary" field is at the moment limited to 5000 characters per citation (dBase III+ text editor limit) which seems adequate but this can easily be changed to involve the WordStar 2000 word processor allowing unlimited summary size.

Search

The function can search and identify all references with any combination of key word(s), journal, author(s), word(s) in title and manual filing number for research purposes. The list of searched references can also be viewed on screen or may be printed out.

The speed of search depends on the size of the reference database, the number of citations that match the search citation and the number of boolean operators used (Fig. 19.5). Any search data can be saved on hard or floppy disc and recalled for later use. In addition, the search can be instructed to retrieve only those articles entered since the previous search.

Delete Record(s)

This is used in conjunction with the search function allowing the user to delete individual references from the searched file. Therefore, the delete record(s) function allows the user to remove references that are not to be printed.

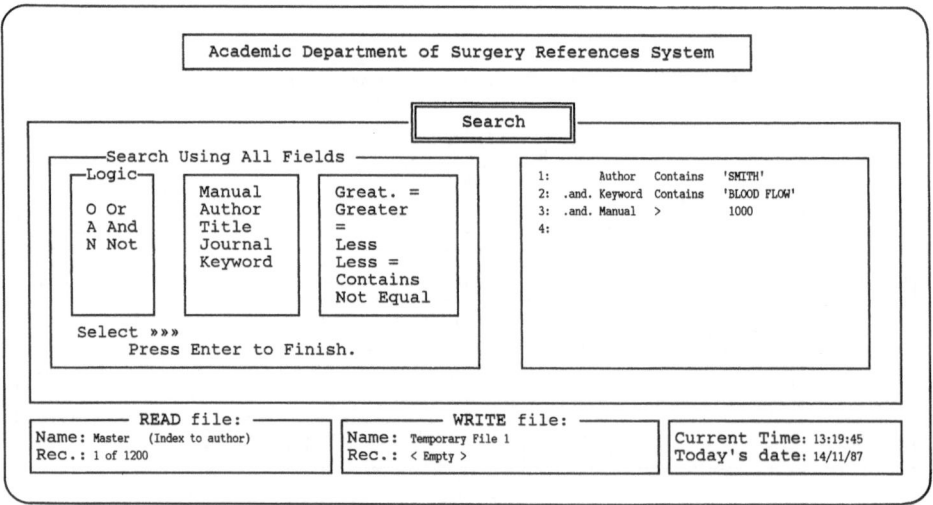

Fig. 19.5. Display of search menu.

Index

The main reference file or any temporary files can be indexed alphabetically by author, title or manual filing number. This option allows the user to select which index style he/she wants and this will be indicated on the bottom of the menu.

Print

The package is interrelated with the WordStar 2000 (R) word processor system. We use dBase to write a file in WordStar's MailMerge data format and then use the word processor program to edit the entry and add it to the document. We have stored a file in the computer describing the Vancouver reference system (International Committee of Medical Journal Editors, 1982) to enable dBase to produce files in the correct style. Only the selected reference can be printed out in the chosen format. Thus the print command requires two selections: one is the name of the database file and the second is the name of the print format to be used.

Change File

At present there are three database files set up. The main one is the master file containing all the references and the other two are temporary files. By using the change file function key it is possible the select files to "read from" and files to "write to". This is used mainly when performing searches. It is possible to increase the number of temporary or master files. Files could be added for each staff member.

Back-up file

This command allows transfer of a selected search or the entire database on a floppy disc for future use, either as a back-up to the hard disc storage or for transporting data to another computer. At present the back-up is done on floppy discs and the speed depends on the number of references. However, we are aiming for a high-capacity disc subsystem with streaming tape back-up for faster response of about 5 Mbyte per minute.

Load File

This allows database files stored on a floppy disc to be loaded on to a Winchester disc and used as needed.

Exit

Quit the reference system.

Reliability

For simplicity, all data should be entered in a consistent manner. A standard style for entering authors' names, reference listing, and key words should be decided upon by the user prior to the first data entry. The reason for this is the limitation of the search. For example, if one of the authors' names, "Alex B. Smith," is entered as (1) Smith, AB, or (2) Smith, A.B., searching by "Smith, A.B." will pick up the second entry only. This problem can be overcome by searching by "Smith"; this will pick up all references whose authors are "Smith". Further searches could then be performed on this reduced database (by using the Change File function key to select the appropriate read, write files) or to use the delete records function key to remove unwanted references. In designing the data entry protocol, spelling, spaces, periods, and commas must be taken into account. Sloppily entered data will result in a decreased output during retrieval.

Conclusion

The program allows the user to store the bibliographic information, as well as any key words or summary information that the user wishes to include. In addition, it permits a rapid computer search for standard scientific articles, using the author(s) name, specific words in the title, key words or journal. The program allows for selected references to be printed subsequently in any format the user specifies. The hierarchical menu-driven system ensures against loss or corruption of any data and provides a user friendly Man–Machine interface.

Further Development

We are in progress of improving the computerised references system further by introducing a mini-dictionary allowing the names of specific journals to be stored without the need to type the name of each in full. This will reduce the typing errors that may arise and ease the data entry. Further improvements will include: checking and eliminating double entry citations and setting up a local area network in the department, which will allow ready access to the system by different staff members.

References

Hunter TB (1983) Simple interactive computer program to store literature references. AJR 140: 169
Kunin CM (1985) Managing bibliographic citations using microcomputers. JAMA 78: 627–634
International Committee of Medical Journal Editors (1982) Style matters: uniform requirements for manuscripts submitted to biomedical journals. Br Med J 284: 1766–1770

20 Using Student Projects to Develop Materials for Children with Special Educational Needs – Experience at Sunderland Polytechnic

C. Bloor

Introduction

At Sunderland Polytechnic we run two main computing degree courses: the BA Business Computing and the BSc Combined Studies in Science. In addition there is a part-time Master's degree in Computer-Based Information Systems, and a part-time BA in Information Technology. All these degrees require that the student complete a project of 70–150 hours duration, giving the lecturing staff the problem of devising approximately 100 projects each year. This paper describes our experience in using student projects to develop material for children with special educational needs in schools contacted via either the Newcastle SEMERC (Special Education Microelectronics Resource Centre) or existing contacts.

The Project

The aim of the project is "To place the student within the constraints of a project format and provide an opportunity for the expression of his or her individual energy and ability in completing a significant item of work in the information systems field."

Generally projects are suggested by lecturing staff and are derived from their research interests, departmental teaching and administration requirements or to simulate "real" systems.

Great emphasis is placed on the management of the project, especially for the Business Computing degree. These students will shortly be entering an industry where the delivery of a correctly functioning product, to budget and on time is all-important. Projects derived from the above sources allow the student to demonstrate management skills but can lack a sense of realness. If the project product is not to be used live, or is intended only for internal consumption, then the student can demonstrate competence by fully analysing and designing a system, and implementing a small part of that system as a prototype or model.

Over the past three years we have worked with the Newcastle SEMERC and other contacts in the locality and have used project students to develop teaching materials for use with SEN (Special Educational Needs) children. All these projects have been successful from the points of view of both the project sponsor and the student. Our students respond to this type of project for a number of reasons.

1. The product is to be a real system for an outside organisation. This makes the production of a working system important and thus adds to the student's motivation
2. The commitment which many students have to help others is exploited
3. The student, having been the receiver in the educational process for a number of years, is able to act as an expert guiding what will be, in many cases, a naive user
4. There is no doubt that this type of project gives ample scope for students to use their own ideas and to demonstrate their energy and abilities. As a prime example of this see 't-Island' which is described below

These projects also have advantages for the sponsors.

1. It is an opportunity for the sponsor to develop his own ideas without the chore of having to learn a programming language
2. This is a two-way process and we would expect the sponsor to learn from our students
3. The sponsor gets access to all the resources of the Polytechnic. We would expect a student to use whatever resources were available, both hardware and staff time, in order to complete the project
4. No expense is involved

Projects Implemented

The following sections give brief descriptions of the projects implemented to date.

Sounds

These programs use speech digitising/playback equipment on the BBC micro and are designed for auditory discrimination work with hearing impaired children. There is a basic "speak and spell" program in which a sentence is displayed on the screen with one word missing. The child has to listen to a recording of the sentence and, using context and aural clues, insert the correct word. There is also a game program in which nine pictures are displayed, in turn, and a sound associated with the picture played. The pictures are then placed in boxes on the screen and the sounds replayed at random. The idea is to guess which picture is related to the sound currently being played. The speech digitiser used is a relatively cheap device but the sound quality produced is good, equivalent in standard to that produced by a cheap tape recorder. Utilities are provided to allow teachers to create their own pictures and to record new sounds.

t-Island

t-Island is an adventure game in which the user has to navigate his way round an island looking for members of his orchestra who have been shipwrecked. The orchestra members are never seen; they are detected by the user hearing the tune they are playing and distinguishing this tune from a different one played by "wicked" musicians trying to get into the orchestra. The program idea was entirely that of the student involved. It was designed for auditory discrimination work with hearing-impaired children but is equally valid for use with normal children. The program develops skills, such as devising strategies which are required for other adventure games. Concepts of direction and map-reading skills are also developed.

Both t-Island (Bloor and Adams 1986) and Sounds (Bloor 1986) have been reported elsewhere.

Ghost Hunt

Positions of objects cause problems for hearing-impaired children who may not appreciate the subtle differences between expressions such as "near to", "next to" and "to the left of", or between "above" and "on top of" etc. At a greater degree of hearing loss the child might be struggling merely to recognise the words of the objects involved, without going to the deeper level of understanding the relationship between the objects. Ghost Hunt was developed as a student project for use with children in a Junior School Partially Hearing Unit. The user moves through a house trying to identify objects whose initial letters form the name of a ghost. Having identified the object the user then has to state its position (from a choice of three), and its colour. Answers are scored with a high score scaring the ghost away as a "reward".

As part of the evaluation of this project the program was used in two main-stream junior schools with normal children, and with children in a remedial learning group. Teachers' comments were favourable in both cases, although for the group of hearing children the age range for which the program was felt to be applicable was lower. This is to be expected, given the retarded language development of hearing-impaired children.

Early Language Work

One of the problems with some commercial software is that once the program has been used a number of times the users become familiar with the program and it loses some of its educational value. This particular set of programs was written for a remedial language unit in a junior school. These programs teach the concepts of "on" and "under" as well as simple sentence construction. The concept keyboard is used. This is an A4 pad with an 8 × 16 array of micro switches under the surface. It is possible to detect the depression of individual switches, or a group of switches. By overlaying the pad with a picture or set of instructions the child is able to point to the desired input. This eliminates the need for keyboard skills in operating the computer.

The principle of the program is that a prompt on the screen asks the child to perform some action. At the initial stage this is just to move one object so that it is either ON or UNDER a second object. The child has to press the right word in order to obtain an animated display of this action performed on the screen. The prompt increases in complexity under the control of the teacher, so that at the highest level the child is presented with several objects. The child has to press the correct words but also in the correct order to obtain the animation. Thus simple sentence construction is taught.

In order to extend the applicability of this program the teacher is provided with a utility which allows new objects to be created and named. The movement on screen, in terms of the start and finish positions in the animation, can also be defined.

In-On-Under and Big-Little

These programs, and those described below, were developed for reception-class children in a school for severely mentally and physically handicapped children. The concepts of "In", "On" and "Under" are taught together with their Bliss Symbols. The Bliss Symbol is displayed to indicate the correct response. An object (man, dog or cat) is then placed in, on, and under a second object in random order. When there is a correct match between the position of the objects and the symbol the child indicates this by pressing a two-way switch or depressing the return key. The teacher can control the number of concepts taught, the number of chances allowed, and the time delay before moving on to the next position. The program also collects statistics on the child's responses. The reward/punishment is the Bliss Symbol for "happy" or "sad".

Big-Little operates in a similar fashion to In-On-Under. The trainee has to match an object (man, child, mouse) with the correctly sized space (door or mousehole). With a correct response the object moves into the space. An incorrect response causes the object to stamp its foot.

Early Learning

These programs aim to enhance motor skills, recognition, vocalisation and concentration skills. By pressing the concept keyboard the child is able to build up a series of clearly recognisable pictures. On completion a short jingle is played. Younger children get enough reward from the program by producing the picture. Older children are motivated by trying to guess what the completed picture will be.

Total Communication Workstation (TCW)

Total communication is a philosophy for the teaching of the profoundly deaf (Evans 1982). It is employed in approximately 8% of the schools and units for hearing-impaired children in the UK (Kunsang 1987). The philosophy is to use any means of communication in order to overcome the very real problems which these children have. Conventionally these communication modes will include speech, sign, gesture, finger spelling and lip-reading. Kingham et al. (1987) have transferred this philosophy to the computer by using:

Graphics to display an animated example of the word being trained together with the British Sign Language (BSL) for that word

Text to give the word in English

Speech recording to give an example of the correct pronunciation of the word

Speech recognition to test the user's utterance

The mode of operation of the workstation is that the teacher would first select the words to be trained, and the communication modes to be used. The trainee is then presented with the text and appropriate graphics. After hearing the prerecorded example of the word the trainee makes his or her response. This is evaluated by the speech recognition equipment, and a reward or punishment given.

The equipment used is an IBM PC or PC-compatible micro and the VOTAN VPC 2000 voice card. The latter is a template matching voice recognition system which also has facilities to record sounds. As this is a template matching system a template, or example of each word which is in the expected vocabulary, has to be collected. The system then recognises sounds by choosing the word in its vocabulary which closest matches the sound uttered. The system may be used in two modes. In wrap-round mode the voice card sits alongside the application program, recognising and passing character strings to the operating system as an alternative to, or in addition to, the keyboard. In VPC mode the command language of the voice card is used to create applications. The latter mode has been used in the TCW. The computational ability of VPL is limited so this is only used to control the speech functions of template collection, speech recording or playback, and actual recognition. The main routines are written in the "C" programming language. Both C and VPL programs run concurrently, communicating via a buffer controlled by the voice card.

The technology used creates two problems. Firstly, the templates have to be collected. If we use the trainee's voice for this we will, in effect, be reinforcing any bad habits of pronunciation which the trainee has. If, on the other hand, we use a teacher's voice, the trainee's efforts may be so far away from that voice as to make the recognition score obtained meaningless. This leads into the problem of scoring the trainee's response. The voice card returns a score of between 0 and 255. 0 is a perfect match. We have overcome this problem in the prototype workstation by setting an initial acceptance level. If the trainee is successful this level is reset to require a better effort next time. If the trainee is unsuccessful, however, the acceptance level is reset to give a "success' with a poorer match. In this way it is hoped that the trainee will receive the stimulus of a correct score, perhaps even with the merest "grunt", and this will encourage a better attempt.

It is intended to extend this project from the prototype stage, and to investigate further a number of issues. At present the VOTAN VPC 2000 is being used in single word mode. The card can recognise continuous speech. This adds a new dimension to the use of the TCW in that in this mode it could be used to teach language rather than isolated words. One can imagine a simple natural language interface in which the user could enquire "Where's the ball?" and receive a response "Here's the ball", with appropriate graphics. There is an obvious need to explore such possibilities in schools and units for hearing-impaired children. Another possible use is in therapy for stroke victims, and for use with the adult mentally handicapped. In the latter case it is presumed that Makatron symbols, rather than BSL, would be employed.

The work has been carried out as part of ESPRIT Project 449, "Investigation into the effective use of speech at the human–machine interface" (ESPRIT 1986). The project was undertaken by a consortium of Voice Systems International Ltd., ICL Defence Systems, Fincantieri and British Maritime Technology Ltd. (BMT). BMT was the main contractor and was responsible for investigating the social benefit of the technology.

Program Development

The TCW was developed and specified by a research student who is also a computing graduate. This is atypical, and many of our project sponsors have been "naive" users unsure of the capabilities of the computer. They are also unsure of how to specify what it is that they do want. The students, too, will not be expert in the BBC machine or its graphics capability. Part of the project is for them to come to grips with a new machine. In these circumstances it is not possible, or desirable, to specify the whole program in one step so a prototyping approach has generally been taken (Martin 1982). The idea is to implement part of the system as a demonstration for the user, or to use "quick and dirty" methods to produce a working model which can then be refined.

Typically the development process might go through the following three stages.

After an initial meeting with the sponsor the student will draw up a narrative account of the system to be developed. This will include rough screen designs. At the next meeting the student and sponsor go through this narrative together. The objective is to get the program specification correct, including the screen designs and any dialogue between the child and computer. There might be major changes requested by the sponsor at this stage.

Having obtained the sponsor's agreement to the paper model of the system one would expect the student to implement one or two of the screens so that at the next meeting the sponsor can go through the paper model working with the actual screens. This stage is generally a major learning step for the student who will not have a great deal of experience of the use of graphics. One of the advantages of prototyping is that the development of part of the system allows better estimates to be made of the financial and time costs for the whole system. At the end of this stage both sponsor and student will have a reasonable idea what can be implemented in the time-scale. This may result in modifications to the system or a decision to implement part of the system only. The sponsor, if a naive user, may not appreciate the graphics capability of the micro being used. It is thus important to agree on the level of sophistication required and to have this demonstrated by the drawing of example screens. The screens implemented will show the sponsor what is practical in terms of colour and resolution with the machine chosen.

The student will now have enough information and expertise fully to implement part of the system. For example, in Ghost Hunt, the search for two articles in one room of the house plus the program introduction was completed at this stage, and demonstrated to the sponsor. One would expect any modifications to be minor and the student to be able to go ahead and implement the whole system.

Conclusions

The response to these projects has been positive, from both the students and sponsors. As a measure of the student's commitment two of these projects (t-island and the TCW prototype) have been awarded the "best project" prize for their course. Sponsors, too, are generally enthusiastic about the final product. The high degree of sponsor involvement at the design stage may be responsible for this. One planned project is to evaluate these programs with other users in other schools.

Acknowledgements. The author would like to acknowledge the enthusiastic contribution made by the following students: Tony Adams, Glen Cook, Les Baker, Vickie Challis, Hazel Fix, and Diane Mitchell. The contribution of project supervisors at Sunderland Polytechnic is also acknowledged, as is the contribution of Mr. L. O. Kingham and Mr. J. L. McCullough to the development of the Total Communication Workstation.

References

Bloor C, Adams T (1986) Computer sounds and hearing impaired children. CET Newsletter: Microelectronics and children with special educational needs. October 1986
Bloor C (1986) The use of microcomputers in the auditory training of hearing impaired children. J Br Assoc Teachers of the Deaf 5: 117–120
ESPRIT (1986) Project 449: Investigation into the effective use of speech at the Human–Machine interface. Public Domain Report. British Maritime Technology, Wallsend Research Station, Tyne and Wear
Evans L (1982) Total Communication: Structure and Strategy. Gallaudet College Press, Washington
Kingham LO, Harris PR, Tolmie IM (1987) The integration of speech technology and graphics as an aid for the disabled. In: Laver J, Jack MA (eds.) European conference on speech technology. CEP Consultants, 26–28 Albany Street, Edinburgh EH1 3QH, pp 339–343
Kunsang M (1987) The 1981 Education Act – a survey of effects on policy and provision for hearing-impaired pupils in the ordinary school. J Br Assoc Teachers of the Deaf 4: 109–118
Martin J (1982) Application Development without programmers. Prentice Hall, Englewood Cliffs, New Jersey

Subject Index